This is a concise, accessible introduction to the essentials of anesthesia, suitable for medical students, junior doctors and all operating theater staff. It provides a brief, broad overview of the science and practice of anesthesia without overwhelming the reader with intimidating detail. The first section of the book describes the evaluation of the patient, the different approaches to anesthesia, and the post-operative care of the patient in pain. The next section introduces the essentials of physiology and pharmacology and their role in understanding the principles of anesthesia. The final section presents a step-by-step description of clinical cases, ranging from the simplest to the most complex. These clinical vignettes give a very real introduction to the practicalities of anesthesia and will give the non-anesthetist physician an idea of how to prepare a patient for a surgical procedure.

Dr. Tammy Euliano, Associate Professor of Anesthesiology, received her M.D. from the University of Florida and continued there throughout residency and fellowship. She has received numerous awards for her dedication to teaching including the International Anesthesia Research Society Teaching Recognition Award (finalist), the University of Florida College of Medicine Exemplary Teacher, and is a member of the Society of Teaching Scholars. Her research in simulator technology and patient safety has also been recognized by the American Society of Anesthesiologists.

Dr. J. S. Gravenstein is Graduate Research Professor of Anesthesiology, Emeritus, University of Florida College of Medicine. Dr. Gravenstein received his Dr. med. from the University of Bonn in Germany and his M.D. from Harvard University School of Medicine. Dr. Gravenstein is known worldwide for his work in patient monitoring, patient safety, and simulation technology. His numerous awards include the Massachusetts General Hospital Trustees' Medal, and an honorary doctorate in medicine from the University of Graz, Austria.

Essential Anesthesia

From Science to Practice

T. Y. Euliano and
J. S. Gravenstein

University of Florida
College of Medicine,
Gainesville, Florida, USA

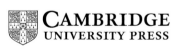
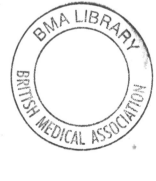
CAMBRIDGE
UNIVERSITY PRESS

PUBLISHED BY THE PRESS SYNDICATE OF THE UNIVERSITY OF CAMBRIDGE
The Pitt Building, Trumpington Street, Cambridge, United Kingdom

CAMBRIDGE UNIVERSITY PRESS
The Edinburgh Building, Cambridge, CB2 2RU, UK
40 West 20th Street, New York, NY 10011–4211, USA
477 Williamstown Road, Port Melbourne, VIC 3207, Australia
Ruiz de Alarcón 13, 28014 Madrid, Spain
Dock House, The Waterfront, Cape Town 8001, South Africa

http://www.cambridge.org

First published 2004

Printed in the United Kingdom at the University Press, Cambridge

Typefaces Utopia 9/13 pt. and Dax   *System* LaTeX 2$_\varepsilon$ [TB]

A catalog record for this book is available from the British Library

Library of Congress Cataloging in Publication data
Euliano, Tammy, 1966–
Essential anesthesia / Tammy Euliano, J. S. Gravenstein.
    p.   cm.
Includes bibliographical references and index.
ISBN 0 521 53600 6 (paperback)
1. Anesthesiology.   2. Anesthesia.   I. Gravenstein, J. S.   II. Title.
RD81.E83   2004
617.9′6–dc22   2004051801

ISBN 0 521 53600 6 paperback

For Alix and Neil

Contents

Foreword

The most recognizable part of the anesthesiologist's work consists of maintaining the stability of the patient's multiple and complex organ systems during surgical operations while providing freedom from pain. To accomplish these sometimes opposing goals, the anesthesiologist must have detailed knowledge of the diseases affecting the patient and must be able to base all therapeutic decisions on an astute understanding of physiology and pharmacology. Emphasizing the serious nature of the anesthetic state, anesthesia has been described as "a controlled overdose of drugs requiring continuous intensive care of the patient." Understandably then, many founders of critical care medicine were anesthesiologists and, by the same token, much material in this book is immediately applicable to the intensive care of critically ill patients.

The authors had set out to write a book to introduce medical students to the complexities of anesthetic practice including compassionate pre- and post-operative care. However, this little book rapidly grew beyond that early goal. Physicians and nurses outside of anesthesia will discover in these pages wonderful reviews of physiology and pharmacology and clinical pearls helpful in preparing a patient for anesthesia and surgery. That Drs. Euliano and Gravenstein have a wealth of teaching experience shows on every page. They successfully present very complex subjects in a lively manner and in relatively simple terms. I am confident that the reader will find this text not only thorough but also – how rare for a medical text – pleasant to read. This book offers answers to many questions, while simultaneously stimulating the reader to consult one of the many voluminous specialty texts that provide details, requiring much more space than available in a volume of this size.

Jerome H. Modell, M.D.

In Greek mythology, the night has twin sons, Thanatos (death) and Hypnos (sleep), who carry flaming torches pointing toward the floor, to light a path through the dark. Juan Marín, a Latin American anesthesia pioneer, designed this image to represent anesthesia. He placed a small light between Thanatos and Hypnos indicating the flame of life the anesthesiologist must guard. The upper half of the emblem shows the rising or setting sun of consciousness. The Confederación Latinoamericana de Anestesiología and the Revista Colombiana de Anestesiología have adopted this beautiful emblem, which in the past had been used by the World Federation of Societies of Anaesthesiologists.

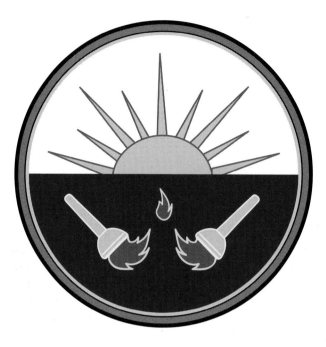

Preface

"What should I read in preparation for a rotation through the anesthesia service?" – so have asked not only students, but also other medical and non-medical visitors to the operating room. In response to this often posed question, we could recommend several wonderful and exhaustive texts, but such tomes demand an investment of time and effort only the dedicated specialist could muster. An introductory text should be easy to read, and it should be short enough to be completed in a few hours. It has to be a sketch instead of a full painting, yet it must clearly show the features of the subject. This we have striven to accomplish but, occasionally, we succumbed and included a bit of trivia. We hope the reader will forgive us for that.

We have divided the little book into three parts. The first part presents the equivalent of a miniature operating manual covering pre-, intra- and post-anesthesia tasks and the tools of the profession. In the second part, we give a synopsis of cardiovascular and respiratory physiology and pharmacology of importance to peri-operative clinical practice. The third part places the reader into the operating room looking over the shoulder of a busy anesthesiologist taking care of patients with special problems. Here, we have chosen common clinical situations, and we have incorporated difficulties – some of them avoidable – in order to highlight challenges faced in daily practice. A reader who had started at the beginning of the book and now looks at the clinical examples should be able to apply much of the information presented in the first and second sections of the book to the problems arising in the clinical cases. Of course, some might prefer to read about the cases first – perhaps in preparation for a visit to the operating room – in order to get a preview of the extraordinary world of clinical anesthesia and surgery. Such an approach should raise many questions in the reader's mind, topics we hope to have touched on in the first two sections of the book.

Our hope is that this little text will intrigue some into further investigation of the fascinating field of anesthesiology, provide insight into the subspecialty for our colleagues in other areas, and improve the understanding of physiology, pharmacology, and peri-operative medicine for all our readers.

T. Y. Euliano, J.S. Gravenstein
July, 2004

Acknowledgements

We are grateful to the many people who helped in the preparation of this text. In particular we thank Dr. Dietrich Gravenstein, Kendra Kuck, Kelly Spaulding, and Frederike Gravenstein for lending their expertise, as well as Peter Silver and Cambridge University Press for providing direction in completing this (first) edition. And finally, we are grateful to the medical students, who prompted the project in the first place, and continue to keep us on our toes.

Introduction
A *very* short history of anesthesia

Every now and then, you run into a high school student who did a paper on the history of anesthesia, or the teacher who assigned it. Here are a few facts and dates that should keep you out of acute embarrassment.

God was first: "And the Lord God caused a deep sleep to fall upon Adam, and he slept." (Genesis 2:21). A date is not given.

Anesthesia as we know it started in the early to mid 1840s.

Crawford Long of Jefferson, Georgia, removed a small tumor from a patient under diethyl ether anesthesia. That was in 1842. Crawford Long failed to publish this event, and he was denied the fame of having been the first to use diethyl ether as a surgical anesthetic. Ether was not unknown; students inhaled it during the so-called ether frolics.

Horace Wells had used nitrous oxide in his dental practice. In 1844, he failed to demonstrate the anesthetic effects of N_2O in front of a critical medical audience. The patient, a boy, screamed during the extraction of a tooth, and the audience hissed. Later, the boy said that he had not felt anything. Excitement under light nitrous oxide anesthesia is common. Horace Wells died young and by his own hand.

William T. G. Morton, another dentist in anesthesia's history, successfully etherized a patient at the Massachusetts General Hospital in Boston on *October 16, 1846*. The news of this event spread worldwide as rapidly as the communication links permitted. Morton tried to patent his discovery under the name of Letheon. An English barrister later wrote: ". . . a patent degrades a noble discovery to the level of a quack medicine."[1]

Oliver Wendell Holmes, only 2 months after Morton's epochal demonstration of surgical anesthesia, suggested the term "anesthesia" to describe the state of sleep induced by ether. Holmes was a physician, poet, humorist and, fittingly, finally dean of Harvard Medical School.

John Snow, from London, became the first physician to devote his energies to anesthetizing patients for surgical operations. His earliest experiences with ether anesthesia date to late 1846. In 1853, he administered chloroform to Queen Victoria for the delivery of her son Prince Leopold. This shook the acceptance of the divine command: "in sorrow thou shalt bring forth children" (Genesis 3:16) and thus powerfully furthered the use of anesthesia to alleviate the pain of childbirth. Incidentally, while anesthesiologists admire John Snow for his publications and the design of an etherizer, epidemiologists claim him as one of their own because he had recognized the source of a cholera epidemic, which he traced to a public pump. By removing the pump's handle, he stopped the spread of the infection. That was in 1854.

Those were the beginnings. By now, the two earliest anesthetic vapors, diethyl ether and chloroform, have been modified hundreds of times. Many descendants have come and gone, but their great-grandchildren still find daily use. Intravenous drugs have secured an increasingly prominent place in anesthesia, among them neuromuscular blockers – hailing back to South American Indians and their poisoned arrows shot from blowguns. A steadily growing pharmacopeia of analgesics, hypnotics, anxiolytics, and cardiovascular drugs now fill the drug cabinets.

We still listen for breath sounds, we still watch color and respiration, and we still feel the pulse, but today we are helped by the most subtle techniques of sensing invisible signals and the most invasive methods with tubes snaking through the heart.

When we reduce the history of anesthesia to a few dates and facts, we do not do justice to the stories of the age-old and arduous struggle to alleviate pain. In one of the more comprehensive books on '*The Genesis of Surgical Anesthesia*', you will find a superb description of the interesting personalities and the many events that eventually paved the way to one of the greatest advances in medicine, the discovery of anesthesia.[2] The book brims with anecdotes, for example the story of a woman in 1591 accused of witchcraft. One of the indictments was for her attempt to ease the pain of childbirth. She was sentenced to be "bund to ane staik and brunt in assis (ashes), quick (alive) to the death". Why society's acceptance of pain relief changed and how obstetrical anesthesia eventually developed is the subject of another great historical book by Donald Caton.[3]

NOTES

1. You will find this quotation in one of the three delightful volumes entitled *Essays of the First Hundred Years of Anaesthesia* by W. Stanley Sykes who relates the most wonderful stories having to do with anesthesia. For example, did you know that to be eaten alive by a lion and the like might not be painful? (Sykes, W.S. (1961). *Essays on the First Hundred Years of Anaesthesia*. Volume 2, pp. 75–79, E&S Livingstone Ltd, Edinburgh.)
2. Norman A. Bergman (1998). Wood Library – Museum of Anesthesiology, Park Ridge, Illinois.
3. Donald Caton (1999). *What a Blessing She had Chloroform*, Yale University Press, New Haven and London.

Part I

Clinical management

Pre-operative evaluation

Surgery and anesthesia cause major perturbations to a patient's homeostasis. The risk of potentially life-threatening complications can be reduced with appropriate pre-operative evaluation and therapy. Because cost concerns have virtually eliminated pre-operative hospital admission, today the visit may occur just moments before the operation in the case of an emergency or a healthy outpatient, but is better managed in pre-anesthesia clinics to which patients report one or several days before their operation. Surgeons and primary-care physicians can do much to avoid operative delays and cancellations, as well as to reduce the patient's cost and risk by identifying patients who need a pre-operative anesthesia consultation and by sending all pertinent information, e.g., recent ECG, echo studies, etc., with the patient. The pre-anesthetic evaluation appears to be just another routine of eliciting a history, reviewing all systems, performing a physical examination, and checking laboratory studies. However, this traditional approach provides the structure that enables us to ferret out information that can affect anesthetic preparation and management. A widely accepted shorthand, the famous ASA Physical Status classification (Table 1.1), summarizes a thorough patient evaluation into a simple scheme, found on every anesthesia record. The six Physical Status classes do *not* address risk specifically, but do provide a common nomenclature when discussing patients in general. That much more than the ASA physical status classification need be known will become apparent from the following.

History

We begin with the "H" in "H&P," obtaining a medical and surgical history. We are particularly concerned with the cardiopulmonary system, and exercise tolerance is a good measure of current status. We also search for evidence of chronic diseases of other systems. For elective procedures, patients should be in the best condition possible, e.g., no exacerbation of chronic bronchitis or unstable angina. Below, we describe the pre-operative evaluation of some common medical conditions. When patients with these, or other rarer, conditions require an anesthetic,

Table 1.1. ASA Physical status classification

I A normal healthy patient
II A patient with mild systemic disease
III A patient with severe systemic disease
IV A patient with severe systemic disease that is a constant threat to life
V A moribund patient who is not expected to survive without the operation
VI A declared brain dead patient whose organs are being removed for donor purposes

We append an "E" if the patient comes in as an emergency.
ASA = American Society of Anesthesiologists

a pre-anesthesia clinic visit a week or so in advance of anesthesia allows time to seek additional information, e.g., study results from the patient's private physician, perform studies, e.g., cardiac pacemaker interrogation, or obtain consultation from a specialist. Such planning helps keep the operating schedule running smoothly.

We inquire about any previous anesthetics, particularly any untoward events such as bleeding or airway difficulties. It is reassuring to learn a patient has tolerated previous anesthetics without difficulties. Next, we ask specifically about any family history of anesthetic complications. A patient might not realize that a remote event, such as his Aunt Edna dying with a raging fever soon after an anesthetic many years ago, might mean that malignant hyperthermia runs in his family. We need to ask specific questions to learn about inherited conditions, including those related to plasma cholinesterase (see Pharmacology: succinylcholine).

Medications

With surprising frequency, review of the patient's current medications reveals previously unmentioned medical problems: "Oh, the digoxin? Well I don't have a heart condition *now*." Many medications influence the anesthetic, particularly those with cardiovascular or coagulation-related effects. Some need to be discontinued for some period prior to surgery (see below), others must be converted from oral to parenteral form to continue their effect. Many patients do not think of herbal compounds when asked about their use of medicines and drugs. Therefore, we need to ask specifically about herbals, some of which may present us with problems.[1]

Allergies

Common are patients with allergies to latex and to drugs. Questions about such sensitivities need to be asked of every patient lest we get confronted with a

Table 1.2. Considerations in the latex-allergic/sensitive patient

Latex-free gloves!
Remove drug vial caps, rather than puncturing the rubber top to draw up drugs.
Confirm latex-free equipment:
    manual breathing bag
    ventilator bellows
    blood pressure cuff
    esophageal/precordial stethoscope tubing
    intravenous tubing access ports
    epidural access port
    syringe plunger caps (LF (latex free) should appear on the top of the plunger).

life-threatening anaphylaxis during anesthesia. A distinction must be made, however, between sensitivities and true allergies. For example, a patient who "thought he was going to die" in the dentist's chair is probably not allergic to local anesthetics; rather, he likely had an intravascular injection, or rapid absorption of epinephrine. Similarly, a patient who gets nauseated from codeine can still receive fentanyl, which is chemically quite different from the morphine-derived drugs. When an allergy is reported to a particular class of drug, there are often other classes available to accomplish the same task. We benefit our patients when we investigate these agents for potential cross-reactivity. For example, a penicillin-allergic patient with a mild reaction in childhood *might* receive a cephalosporin safely (8% cross-reactivity); when determining the risk: benefit ratio, you must take into consideration their reaction and the indication for the cephalosporin.

Latex allergy deserves special mention as its recognition has grown substantially in recent years. The allergy to this natural rubber[2] occurs after repeated exposure (as in the spina bifida patient who must frequently catheterize his bladder). Its sudden rise in healthcare workers coincides with the 1980s admonition of "Universal Precautions" by the US Occupational Safety and Health Administration – healthcare workers were required to wear gloves to prevent transmission of AIDS and other viral illnesses.

While some patients merely note skin irritation from rubber gloves (probably not a real allergy, but a precursor), of great concern is the patient who has experienced throat swelling, for example when blowing up a balloon or painting a room with latex paint. Latex is found in much of our medical equipment – from breathing bags, to syringe plungers, to the puncturable tops on drug vials. In a patient with latex allergy, we must eliminate all latex-containing products from contact with the patient, including indirect contact such as drawing up drugs through a latex plug (Table 1.2).

We mentioned that healthcare workers are at risk. In fact, about one-third will develop a contact dermatitis to latex gloves, while 10% or more may develop a full-blown allergy, even more frequent in those who have other allergies, the so-called atopic individual. We can reduce our risk of developing this allergy by using non-latex gloves, or at least avoiding latex gloves containing cornstarch. While the cornstarch makes the glove easier to don and remove, it solubilizes the latex protein, increasing the chances of making its way through the skin – particularly through skin already irritated by the cornstarch; it also helps the latex protein become aerosolized (and breathed in) upon glove removal.

Habits

Moderate tobacco and alcohol intake are not of great concern, but the chronic alcoholic patient who has experienced delirium tremens, or the smoker who suffers severe pulmonary disease confronts us with serious problems. Patients who take street drugs also challenge us. On the one hand, they may not tell the truth about their habits; on the other hand, if they do take drugs, their response to anesthetics can be quite abnormal and troubling. These street drugs are known by colorful names to some of their devotees. Anesthesia affects the respiratory and cardiovascular systems; therefore, street drugs that depress the CNS can exaggerate respiratory depression, while CNS stimulants such a cocaine can cause fatal cardiac complications.

Physical examination

In addition to the cardiopulmonary examination, we carefully evaluate the patient's airway to predict whether it will be easily intubated (see Airway management). The physical examination should also seek pre-existing neurologic deficits, particularly if regional anesthesia, e.g., spinal, epidural or nerve plexus block, is considered, and any limitations to flexibility that may present difficulties with positioning the patient. If we plan on regional anesthesia, we need to inspect the anatomy, for example, does the patient have a scoliosis that would make a lumbar puncture difficult, or is his skin infected over the site where we would place the needle?

Laboratory evaluations and studies

Here we must ask the question, "Can the results from additional tests influence my anesthetic and post-anesthetic management?" In the majority of cases, the answer turns out to be "No," but there are many exceptions. Among them might be a determination of serum potassium if we fear that the patient is hyperkalemic, in which case a succinylcholine-induced release of potassium would be dangerous.

Coagulation studies would be needed if we plan regional anesthesia and have reason to worry about a bleeding diathesis or thrombocytopenia. Uncontrolled bleeding into the nerve plexus can cause permanent damage. In general, laboratory and other studies should be ordered as indicated from the medical history, and only if they might have an effect on intra- or post-operative management, or perhaps if the risk analysis may suggest canceling or altering the procedure itself. For example, suppose we detect a carotid bruit during the pre-anesthetic evaluation of a patient scheduled for elective hip replacement. While an asymptomatic bruit may not be an indication for operative repair, a significant carotid stenosis may temper our enthusiasm for induced hypotension (intentional blood pressure reduction to reduce intra-operative blood loss).

NPO status

During induction of general anesthesia, the gag reflex is necessarily abolished. Should the patient "choose" that most inopportune time to suffer gastro-esophageal reflux (or worse yet, emesis), there is a high likelihood the stomach contents could end up in the lung, causing a chemical pneumonitis or even acute suffocation from the lodging of solid particles in the bronchial tree. In addition to pharmacologic means (see Pharmacology), we minimize this risk by having the patient report for surgery with an empty stomach. Patients are asked to refrain from eating solid foods for 6–8 hours prior to elective surgery. While there is evidence that clear liquid ingestion is cleared rapidly and not dangerous in those patients with normal digestion (it may even *raise* the pH of the stomach contents above the pH 2.5 danger zone), it remains customary to tell patients who are scheduled for an elective operation in the morning not to eat or drink anything for at least 6 hours (for infants about 2 to 3 hours) before the operation. If the patient is already in the hospital, we write the order "NPO after midnight"[3] to achieve the same results. Here, we can also order "maintenance i.v. fluids" overnight to keep the patient hydrated. Therefore, on the day of surgery we ask every patient about their most recent intake of food and liquids. Avoid asking: "When did you have your last meal?" If the patient's history identifies risk factors for aspiration, e.g., gastroesophageal reflex disease (GERD), diabetes, increased intra-abdominal pressure, hiatal hernia, and requires general anesthesia, we use a rapid sequence induction (see General anesthesia). Pre-operatively, we also consider pharmacologic means to reduce stomach volume and strengthen the lower esophageal sphincter with a prokinetic agent and/or raise gastric pH with H_2 blockers or a proton pump inhibitor.

Many patients have not been fasting for several hours, or their stomach did not have time to empty. Labor pains, narcotics, or trauma can stop gastric peristalsis for hours on end. Of course, in the presence of an ileus, we assume the stomach not to be empty even if the patient had nothing by mouth for many hours or even days.

Planned procedure

The planned surgical, diagnostic, or therapeutic procedure influences the anesthetic management, sometimes producing problems for which we must be prepared. For example, the neurosurgeon may trigger a wild release of catecholamines when destroying the trigeminal ganglion in a percutaneous procedure that lasts only minutes. How are we going to protect the patient from the expected sympathetic storm? Or, how can we guard against a sudden and substantial rise in peripheral arterial resistance when the surgeon clamps the aorta in preparation for the resection of an aortic aneurysm? The planned procedure also has implications for, among other things, intra-operative positioning of the patient, potential need for blood replacement, anticipated severity of post-operative pain (is a regional anesthetic an option?), and need for intensive care after surgery.

Anesthetic choice

In addition to the above assessment, the anesthetic plan must consider the wishes of both patient and surgeon, as well as *our* individual skill and experience. Does the patient have special requests that need to be taken into account? For example, some patients would like to be awake (maybe the President so he doesn't have to pass control of the US to the Vice-President), others asleep, and others do not want "a needle in the back."

Some patients present special problems, for example Jehovah's Witnesses who do not accept blood transfusions, based on their interpretation of several passages in the Bible (for example Acts 15:28, 29). A thoughtful and compassionate discussion with the patient usually finds the physician agreeing to honor the patient's wishes, an agreement that may not be violated. The caring for children of Jehovah's Witnesses brings an added concern and may require ethics consultation and perhaps even referral to a court. Again, these issues are best brought out days prior to surgery at a scheduled pre-anesthetic evaluation.

Numerous studies have failed to demonstrate that a particular inhalation anesthetic, muscle relaxant, or narcotic made for a better outcome than an alternative. Yet, over the years, actual or perceived differences and conveniences have caused some drugs to disappear and others to establish themselves. Given an array of options, we can often consider different approaches to anesthesia, which we can discuss with the patient. We should always recommend the approach with which we have the greatest experience and which we would select for ourselves or a loved one.

The choices depend on several factors, first of which is the surgical procedure. For example, the site of the operation, e.g., a craniotomy, can rule out spinal anesthesia. The nature of the operation, e.g., a thoracotomy, can compel us to use an endotracheal tube. For the removal of a wart or toenail or the lancing of a boil, we would not consider general anesthesia – unless the patient's age or psychological condition would make it preferable. The preferences of the surgeon might also be considered.

This introduces the patient's condition as a factor in the choice of anesthesia. For example, a patient in hemorrhagic shock depends on a functioning sympathetic nervous system for survival and therefore cannot tolerate the sympathetic blockade induced by spinal or epidural anesthesia. A patient with an open eye can lose vitreous if the intra-ocular pressure rises, as might occur with the use of succinylcholine. Vigorous coughing at the end of an eye operation might do the same and must be avoided. Respiratory depression and elevated arterial carbon dioxide levels can increase intracranial pressure with potentially devastating effects in patients with an intracranial mass or hemorrhage. In obstetrical anesthesia, mother *and* child have to be considered. Here, we do not wish to depress uterine contraction nor cause prolonged sedation of the newborn child. Some agents used in anesthesia rely on renal excretion, others on hepatic metabolism, thus tilting our choice of drugs in patients with renal or hepatic insufficiency.

In the majority of patients, however, it makes little difference what we pick. We could choose one or the other technique for general anesthesia, using one or the other intravenous induction drug and neuromuscular blocker, and relying on one or the other inhalation anesthetic. We can supplement such a technique with one of a number of narcotic drugs available to us, or we can use total intravenous anesthesia. When we use general anesthesia, we can intubate the patient's trachea and let the patient breathe spontaneously, or we can artificially ventilate the patient's lungs. Instead of an endotracheal tube, we have available the laryngeal mask airway, preferably used in spontaneously breathing patients or, in the very old-fashioned approach, we might use only a face mask.

In many instances, we have options, the choice of which will be influenced by our own experience and expertise. For example, anesthesiologists with extensive experience in regional anesthesia will select that technique in preference to general anesthesia in cases where either technique can prove satisfactory for patient and surgeon. Examples include many orthopedic operations or procedures on the genitourinary tract.

In summary, many factors can influence the choice of anesthesia. In the majority of patients, however, we have the luxury of making the choice influenced by our own preference and routine (Fig. 1.1).

Fig. 1.1 The diagram shows the factors to be considered in the choice of anesthesia. In many instances the three circles coincide or greatly overlap, in others the choice is narrowed by the listed factors.

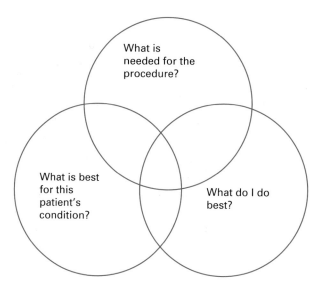

Common disorders

We encounter many patients with pre-existing medical conditions. Anesthetic and operative procedures constitute a physiologic trespass with which the patient can deal better, if not simultaneously challenged by correctable derangements that sap his strength and threaten his homeostasis. Ideally, the surgeon would already have addressed these questions. However, that is not always the case, and the anesthesiologist needs to assess the medical condition of the patient. The answers to the question, "Is the patient in the optimal condition to proceed with anesthesia and operation?" are not always clear-cut. For example, a patient with transient ischemic attacks is scheduled for a carotid endarterectomy. The patient also has coronary artery disease and unstable angina. Should we risk the possibility of a stroke by first putting the patient through a heart operation, or should we risk a myocardial infarction by first doing a carotid endarterectomy? Consultations with other experts help in resolving such difficult issues.

Trauma emergency

Rapid assessment of the airway and fluid status precedes, or coincides with, the most urgent: stemming of hemorrhage. Once we have secured an airway and established a route for administering fluids, we can contemplate anesthesia, realizing that a patient in hemorrhagic shock will tolerate and require very little anesthesia. The mechanism of the trauma may suggest additional studies (Table 1.3).

Table 1.3. Studies in the trauma patient

Study	Indication	Comments
Cervical spine radiographs	Trauma, especially with neck tenderness	Traditional direct laryngoscopy can further compromise the cervical spinal cord
Chest radiograph	Any chest trauma or motor vehicle accident	Potential for pneumothorax (avoid nitrous oxide, consider chest tube); pulmonary contusion
Echocardiography	Direct trauma to chest, for example, forceful contact with steering wheel	Cardiac contusion
Abdominal ultrasound	Direct trauma or motor vehicle accident	Potential for hemorrhage, ruptured spleen; replaces diagnostic peritoneal lavage (DPL)
Angiography	Chest or abdominal trauma	Aortic dissection

Diabetes

We focus on the many end-organ effects of diabetes, as well as the patient's glucose control (HgbA1c). Those with poor control should be considered for pre-admission. Pre-operative studies should include assessment of metabolic, renal, and cardiac status. In general, diabetic patients should be scheduled early in the day.

Because of the 30% incidence of gastroparesis in this population, diabetics are often pretreated with metoclopramide to speed gastric emptying and are induced with a 'rapid sequence induction' (see General anesthesia). Intra-operative management aims to match insulin requirements, recognizing the fasting state and the effects of surgical stress.

Coronary artery disease

In 2002, the American College of Cardiology and the American Heart Association (ACC/AHA) published updated guidelines for the perioperative cardiovascular evaluation of patients for non-cardiac surgery. These so-called "Eagle criteria" should be applied only when the results are likely to impact care. We should always ask the patient about their exercise tolerance; the ACC/AHA recommendations attempt to quantify this by using metabolic equivalents (METs), which enables us to classify patients on a scale of 1 (take care of yourself around the house) to 10+ (participate in strenuous sports). A useful dividing line is 4 METs (climb a flight of stairs). In general, patients unable to do more than 4 METs represent a group at high risk of cardiovascular complications. The algorithm in Fig. 1.2 helps in assigning risks and identifying those patients who require additional cardiac evaluation. In addition to their functional capacity, the algorithm incorporates medical status (Table 1.4) and the procedure planned (Table 1.5).

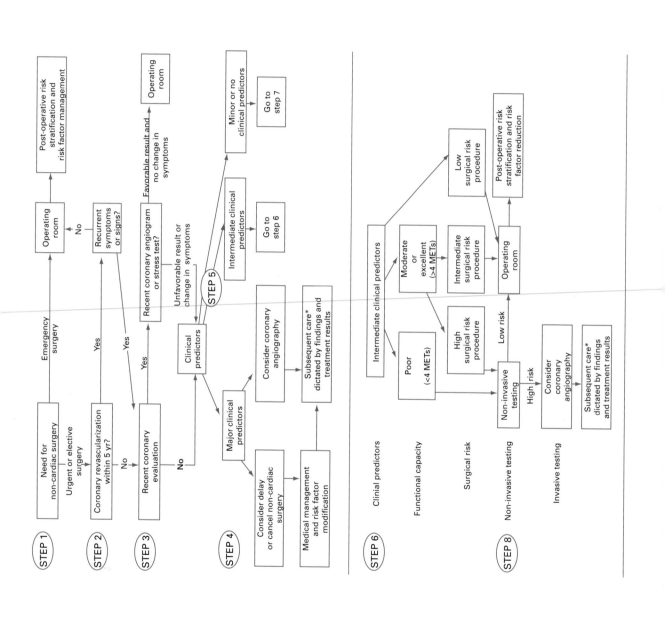

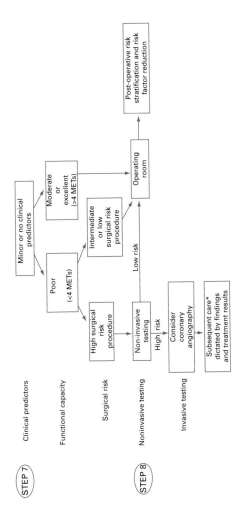

Fig. 1.2 ACC/AHA Guidelines for the perioperative cardiovascular evaluation for noncardiac surgery. A stepwise approach to the risk assessment of patients with pre-existing cardiac disease, scheduled for surgery. Clinical predictors refer to Table 1.4. *Subsequent care may include cancellation or delay of surgery, coronary revascularization followed by noncardiac surgery, or intensified care. (Reproduced with permission from *J Am Coll Cardiol* 1996;27:910–48. Copyright 1996 The ACC Foundation and AHA, Inc. Permission granted for one time use. Further reproduction is not permitted without permission of the ACC/AHA.)

Table 1.4. Clinical predictors of increased perioperative cardiovascular risk (myocardial infarction, heart failure, death)

Major
- Unstable coronary syndromes
- Decompensated heart failure
- Significant arrhythmias
- Severe valvular disease

Intermediate
- Mild angina pectoris
- Previous myocardial infarction
- Compensated or prior heart failure
- Diabetes mellitus (particularly insulin-dependent)
- Renal insufficiency

Minor
- Advanced age
- Abnormal ECG (left ventricular hypertrophy, left bundle-branch block, ST-T abnormalities)
- Rhythm other than sinus
- Low functional capacity, e.g., inability to climb one flight of stairs with a bag of groceries
- History of stroke
- Uncontrolled systemic hypertension

Table 1.5. Cardiac risk[a] stratification for non-cardiac surgical procedures

High (Reported cardiac risk often greater than 5%)
- Emergent major operations, particularly in the elderly
- Aortic and other major vascular surgery
- Peripheral vascular surgery
- Anticipated prolonged surgical procedures associated with large fluid shifts and/or blood loss

Intermediate (Reported cardiac risk generally less than 5%)
- Carotid endarterectomy
- Head and neck surgery
- Intraperitoneal and intrathoracic surgery
- Orthopedic surgery
- Prostate surgery

Low (Reported cardiac risk generally less than 1%)
- Endoscopic procedures
- Superficial procedures
- Cataract surgery
- Breast surgery

[a] Combined incidence of cardiac death and non-fatal myocardial infarction.

Table 1.6. Pacemaker generators

Cardiac chamber paced	Cardiac chamber sensed	Response to sensed R and P
V-Ventricle	V-Ventricle	T-Triggering
A-Atrium	A-Atrium	I-Inhibited
D-Dual	D-Dual	D-Dual
	O-None (asynch)	O-None (asynch)

VVI: Stimulation and sensing occurs in the ventricle. "I" indicates that the pacemaker does not fire if it detects a native R wave. Depending on the patient's intrinsic heart rate, an ECG will show either ventricular pacing or no pacing.
VVIR: As above but responds to patient motion by increasing heart rate. Shivering or fasciculations may erroneously cause an increased pacing rate.
DDD: Stimulates atrium and ventricle, senses P and R waves.
VOO: Asynchronous ventricular pacing. This can cause a problem if a paced R wave occurs during the T wave of a native beat (R-on-T phenomenon).

Pacemaker/AICD

Pacemakers are life saving for many patients with heart rhythm disturbances. There are many types available, with a range of functionality (see Table 1.6). The addition of an automatic internal cardiac defibrillator goes one step further. Unfortunately, these life-saving devices may fail to function properly in the presence of electrical devices, e.g., electrocautery. Many patients carry a card identifying the pacemaker make and model. Some can also provide a report from a recent electronic interrogation that specifies proper function and remaining battery life. More often than not, we do not have that information. A chest radiograph can reveal pacer make and model, as well as lead location. In symptomatic (lightheaded spells, palpitations, hypotension) or in pacer-dependent patients, a pacemaker interrogation (by a specialist with proprietary communication equipment) may be necessary. If this is not an option, a current ECG *might* be helpful, if it demonstrates pacer spikes in appropriate locations.

Pulmonary disease

The patient with pre-operative pulmonary disease faces risks of intra-operative and post-operative pulmonary complications including pneumonia, bronchospasm, atelectasis, respiratory failure with prolonged mechanical ventilation, and exacerbation of pre-existing lung disease. The risk of these complications depends on both the patient and the procedure.

- *Chronic pulmonary disease* Both chronic obstructive pulmonary disease (COPD) and asthma can increase the risk. Therefore, well before anesthesia and surgery we should treat the patient to bring him into the best possible condition, given his lung disease.
- *Smoking* Even without evident lung disease, smoking increases the risk of pulmonary complications up to four times over that or non-smokers. Eight weeks of smoking cessation isf required to reduce that risk, though carboxyhemoglobin will virtually vanish after only 24 smoke-free hours.
- *General health* There are general risk indices that predict pulmonary complications well. In fact, exercise tolerance alone is an excellent predictor of post-operative pulmonary complications.
- *Obesity* Obese patients present more airway management difficulties for several reasons: (i) mechanical issues related to optimal positioning; (ii) redundant pharyngeal tissue complicating laryngoscopy; (iii) many suffer from obstructive sleep apnea (and its sequelae: pulmonary hypertension/cor pulmonale); and (iv) in obese patients it can be extremely difficult or impossible to mask–ventilate the lungs due to the weight of the chest wall. Obesity also increases the risk for thromboembolic phenomena. Post-operatively, however, obesity has not proven to increase the risk of pulmonary complications.
- *Surgical site* Proximity of the surgical site to the diaphragm is the single most important predictor of pulmonary complications. Thoracic and upper abdominal operative sites confer a 10–40% incidence. This can be reduced perhaps 100-fold with laparoscopic techniques.
- *Surgery duration* Operations lasting <3 hours are associated with fewer complications.
- *Intra-operative muscle relaxants* Pancuronium, specifically, has been associated with an increased incidence of pulmonary complications; this is related to its long half-life and risk of residual muscle weakness.
- *Results of pre-operative testing* Routine pre-operative pulmonary function tests (PFTs) are not indicated, unless the patient is undergoing lung resection. If available, however, the risk of complications increases when the forced expiratory volume in 1s (FEV_1) or forced vital capacity (FVC) are <70% predicted, or when the FEV_1/FVC is <65%.

Asthma

Pre-operatively, our goals are to reverse bronchospasm and inflammation, prevent an asthma exacerbation, clear secretions, and treat any infection. We specifically ask about any increased inhaler use, recent hospitalizations or Emergency Department visits for bronchospasm, a recent change in sputum amount or color, or a recent cold. All of these factors increase the risk of peri-operative bronchospasm. If the patient is scheduled for thoracic or upper abdominal surgery (with a very high risk of pulmonary complications), spirometry can identify patients at greatest risk.

Glucocorticoids may be helpful in those patients who do not respond adequately to β_2 agonists. Patients who are steroid dependent will often have suppressed adrenal cortical function and require supplemental steroids in the peri-operative period.

Chronic renal failure

Chronic renal failure (CRF) involves both the excretory and synthetic functions of the kidney. When the kidney fails to regulate fluids and electrolytes, the net result is acidosis, hyperkalemia, hypertension, and edema. Meanwhile, the lack of synthetic function results in anemia (due to decreased production of erythropoietin) and hypocalcemia from a lack of active vitamin D_3 (this also leads to secondary hyperparathyroidism, hyperphosphatemia, and renal osteodystrophy). Azotemia can cause platelet dysfunction.

Medications that are renally excreted will be affected by CRF, and most should be avoided. In particular, meperidine (pethidine, Demerol®) should not be given as its metabolite (normeperidine) can accumulate and cause seizures. The preferred muscle relaxant is one that does not depend on renal function for its metabolism (atracurium, *cis*-atracurium for surgical relaxation).

We check electrolytes on these patients pre-operatively and prefer they undergo dialysis within the preceding 24 hours. We must resist the temptation to hydrate a patient who is intravascularly 'dry' following dialysis, as they cannot excrete excess fluids. Replacement fluids should not contain potassium (normal saline is preferred over Ringer's lactate) as these patients are at risk for hyperkalemia. CRF patients are also at increased risk for coronary artery and peripheral vascular disease.

Pre-operative medication management

Peri-operative beta blockade

The last few years have seen increasing interest in the prophylactic use of beta-blockade to reduce peri-operative cardiac morbidity, particularly in patients at high risk for a cardiac event and undergoing major elective non-cardiac surgery. The target of this therapy is a heart rate of 70 beats/min and systolic BP of 110 mmHg – if tolerated by the patient. If the patient is not currently on beta-blockers, a cardioselective agent (atenolol or metoprolol) is recommended. Unless contraindicated, this blockade should be initiated *as early as possible* and maintained throughout the hospitalization and after discharge (at least 30 days and probably longer).

Antihypertensives

Angiotensin-converting enzyme (ACE) inhibitors (and angiotensin II antagonists) have been linked to severe and refractory intra-operative hypotension under anesthesia. Unless the patient has very severe hypertension, many recommend discontinuation of these medications the day before surgery. Similarly, many advocate discontinuing diuretics the morning of surgery, both for the patient's comfort (if awake) and for intra-operative fluid management. If the diuretic is for acute CHF, however, it should be continued. Otherwise, antihypertensive drugs should be continued the morning of surgery. In particular, agents with a known rebound phenomenon, i.e., clonidine and beta-blockers, *must* be continued or refractory hypertension may result. Because patients are instructed to be fasting, we must actually *tell* them to take their antihypertensives or risk significant hypertension in the pre-operative holding area.

Anticoagulants

Many patients are on some form of platelet inhibitors. While single agent therapy poses no problem for most operations, multi-modal platelet inhibition may increase the risk of peri-operative bleeding.

- *Non-steroidal anti-inflammatory agents (NSAIDs, including aspirin (ASA))* These can be safely continued unless there are special surgical (aesthetic plastic surgery, neurosurgery) or anesthetic (nerve block) considerations, or the patient is on multi-modal therapy. Many surgeons, however, want ASA discontinued 2 weeks prior to surgery and other NSAIDs stopped for at least several days, even though we lack evidence that this alters the incidence of intra-operative blood loss. Actually, it may increase the incidence of thrombotic complications (deep vein thrombosis (DVT), coronary thrombosis, thrombotic stroke), and prevent the pre-emptive analgesia and opioid-sparing capacity of pre-operative NSAIDs.
- *Platelet-function inhibitors (ticlopidine (Ticlid®), clopidogrel (Plavix®))* If the patient receives multi-modal therapy, consider switching to a single agent. We must weigh the risks of discontinuing anticoagulation, with the risk of intra-operative or anesthetic-induced bleeding. Because of their prolonged half-lives, regional anesthesia would mandate discontinuing these agents many days (ticlopidine: 10–14 days; clopidogrel: 7 days) prior to surgery.
- *GP IIb IIIa inhibitors (abciximab (Reopro®), eptifibatide (Integrilin®), tirofiban (Aggrastat®))* These should be stopped prior to surgery and can be reversed with transfusion of platelets. However, patients on these agents usually *need* the anticoagulation. These drugs represent a contraindication to regional anesthesia.

- *Heparin* Subcutaneous prophylactic dosing probably need not be discontinued unless a regional anesthetic is to be administered (4 h), but Lovenox® (low molecular weight heparin) should be stopped 12 h before surgery.

Monoamine oxidase inhibitors (MAOIs)

These agents interact with many drugs and may result in severe hypertension if indirect-acting vasopressors are administered. Even more worrisome are excitatory/depressive (central serotonin syndrome) reactions with administration of opioids. In particular, meperidine (Demerol®) is absolutely contraindicated in these patients. Some still advocate discontinuation of these agents for 2 weeks pre-operatively.

Herbal remedies

Public enthusiasm for herbal supplements has its drawbacks. The following are current considerations together with the recommended discontinuation period prior to surgery:
- Ephedra – works like ephedrine with direct and indirect sympathomimetic effects and all the consequent side effects including intra-operative hemodynamic instability from depletion of endogenous catecholamines; 24 h
- Garlic – inhibition of platelet aggregation and increased fibrinolysis; 7 d
- Ginkgo – inhibition of platelet-activating factor; 36 h
- Ginseng – hypoglycemia, inhibition of platelet aggregation; 7 d
- St. John's Wort – induction of cytochrome P450 enzymes; 5 d
- Others are sedatives such as Kava and Valerian, perhaps reducing the need for additional sedative agents – titrate!

Informed consent

Up into the 1950s, anesthesia claimed about one life of every 2000 anesthetics given. Particularly during the last 30 years, the frequency of anesthesia-related complications leading to morbidity and mortality has decreased markedly, but unfortunately not to zero. No one knows the actual incidence of preventable anesthetic deaths; currently quoted numbers range from 1 in 20 000 to 1 in 200 000 anesthetics; a reasonable estimate probably lying somewhere in the middle of these figures.

Anesthetic risks are usually smaller than the risks associated with surgical interventions, but they loom large when general anesthesia or heavy sedation is required for a non-invasive and essentially risk-free diagnostic examination.

For example, when a small child needs anesthesia to hold still for a CT scan or MRI study, anesthesia poses the only risks.

Many drugs used in general anesthesia interfere with ventilation – think of respiratory depression from narcotics, surgical anesthesia depressing reflexes and relaxing the muscles of the upper airway and, worst of all, the commonly used neuromuscular blocking agents, which spare the heart but paralyze the muscles of respiration. Recognition of these potential respiratory problems has led to the widespread use of endotracheal anesthesia, which requires the insertion of a tube into the trachea, another potential for trouble. Tracheal intubation is not always easy, and unrecognized esophageal intubation continues to claim lives. No wonder then that inadequate ventilation and hypoxemia have caused more grief than any other anesthetic complication. No organ depends more on continuous perfusion with oxygen-carrying blood than the brain. The consequences of brain hypoxia range from deterioration of intellectual function to death.

Anesthetics also affect the cardiovascular system by weakening the myocardium, by depressing autonomic control, and by a relaxing effect on smooth vascular muscles. Decreased preload, low cardiac output, and hypotension result with potential disastrous consequences.

Regional anesthesia carries the risks associated with potential local anesthetic toxicity, resulting in hypotension or convulsions. In addition, the injection of drugs into a nerve plexus, a nerve, or into the epidural or subarachnoid space, carries the risk of physical damage, bleeding, and infection. These complications have been known to cause permanent neurologic changes and even paralysis.

Few drugs are free of the potential for triggering an anaphylactic response, which can be difficult to diagnose in a patient under general anesthesia. The resulting severe hypotension and bronchospasm can then threaten the life of the patient.

Anesthetic morbidity is not easily defined but is certainly more common than mortality. Intra-operative hypotension and arrhythmias are common and, unless severe, are not even mentioned as complications. Within hours after general anesthesia, 25% of all patients may experience cognitive dysfunction; fewer suffer from nausea and vomiting and/or sore throat, and even fewer have peripheral nerve impairment, which usually resolves within weeks. Occasionally, we chip a tooth during tracheal intubation, cause a hematoma with an i.v. catheter, or produce more significant complications with invasive monitors, e.g., a pneumothorax with a central catheter.

In short, anesthesia does pose dangers. This raises the question of how to tell a patient about potential complications in anesthesia or other procedures. Should we pat the patient on the back and say, "Don't worry, I'll take care of you"? Or should we enumerate all possible complications? What does the patient need to understand, and what are we legally required to explain? The informed consent process should result in the active participation of an autonomous and competent patient choosing an anesthetic course based on the information and compassionate medical advice. Physicians have been criticized either for being overly paternalistic, or aloof and impersonal. Frequent complaints concern failure to explain findings and/or treatment plans. While it would be ideal for each patient to understand the details of his or her medical care and participate in all decisions, that level of true "informed consent" is unattainable. Patients will almost invariably be cared for by several experts. Even an expert physician in one field cannot fully appreciate the depth of knowledge an expert in another field brings to the table; how much less then can a medically naïve patient hope to understand all ramifications of diagnosis, prognosis, treatment options, and complications?

Informed consent should fulfill both ethical and legal obligations in the physician–patient relationship, including the pros and cons of the anesthetic options and a description of complications with a 10% or greater risk of occurrence. In addition, rarer complications should be discussed if their disclosure might affect the patient's decision whether to proceed or seek alternative therapy. Otherwise, it is ethically preferable and legally sound to ask whether the patient wishes to hear about the less common but more serious risks before presenting a comprehensive and dizzying list. For example, enumerating risks of heart attack, stroke and death from anesthesia, need not further upset a patient who is undergoing a necessary operation. He already knows he could die from the operation itself or from refusing surgery.

When speaking with patients, before asking for their signature on a document entitled "Informed consent," we find ourselves confronted by a multi-horned dilemma. We wish to explain our findings and therapeutic options, realizing that the patient has a right to make decisions about his or her care. While we do not wish to be paternalistic, we have the obligation to offer our opinion as to the best treatment plan so that the patient has the benefit of our knowledge. Sometimes, our opinion can be colored by our personal skills; when two treatments are equivalent in all aspects, we should prefer the one with which we have more experience. The legally required "informed consent" process, therefore, calls for skillful and compassionate blending of information and guidance covering (i) risks, complications and consequences of the proposed treatment, (ii) alternatives, and (iii) conflicts of interest.

NOTES

1. www.anest.ufl.edu/EA.
2. from the *Hevea brasiliensis* tree.
3. NPO stands for Latin *nil per os* = nothing by mouth.

Airway management

We have made remarkable advances in techniques to secure a patent airway, and have developed new equipment and methods to monitor breathing. Yet, respiratory complications remain the leading cause of anesthesia-related deaths, with the majority related to failure to obtain control of the airway. Here we will discuss: (i) how to evaluate the airway of a patient; (ii) the impact of the planned procedure designed to protect the airway; and (iii) how to manage the airway. First, let us explain why all this matters.

Any time we anesthetize a patient, we must be prepared to take over his ventilation at a moment's (or less) notice because anesthesia can interfere with the patient's ventilation in so many ways. We may have weakened, with muscle relaxants, the patient's ability to breathe. We may have put him into a deep coma, anesthetizing his respiratory center and relaxing the muscles in his mouth and pharynx so that his air passage is obstructed. We might have suppressed his urge to breathe with hypnotics and narcotics during nothing more than a minor surgical procedure. Whatever the roots of the failure to breathe, we must be ready to ventilate the patient's lungs, which means establishing or re-establishing a patent airway and, if necessary, breathing for the patient.

Therefore, before anesthetizing any patient, we examine the airway, looking for physical findings that can be reassuring or worrisome.

Examination of the airway

Direct laryngoscopy (see below) requires neck flexibility, a mouth that can open widely, and no excessive pharyngeal tissue or a large tongue to get in the way. These features cannot be measured directly, but the following steps help us to assess problems that might arise during laryngoscopy:

- Assess mouth opening: inter-incisor distance should exceed 4 cm in an adult.
- Determine the mentum–hyoid (>4 cm) or thyromental (>7 cm) distance: shorter distances suggest an anterior or very cephalad larynx, which would be difficult to visualize by laryngoscopy.

Table 2.1. Trauma evaluation of the cervical spine: findings that may compel radiographic assessment

Midline cervical tenderness
Focal neurologic deficit
Decreased alertness
Intoxication
Painful, distracting injuries that might mask neck pain

From Hoffman, J.R., Mower, W.R., *et al.* Validity of a set of clinical criteria to rule out injury to the cervical spine in patients with blunt trauma. *N. Engl. J. Med.* 2000;**343**:94–9.

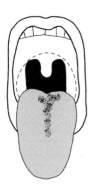 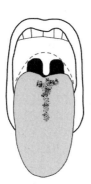 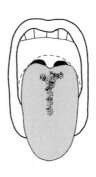 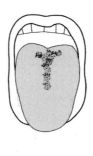

Class I   Class II   Class III   Class IV

Fig. 2.1 Modified Mallampati classification: Class I: soft palate, fauces, uvula, pillars; Class II: soft palate, fauces, portion of uvula; Class III: soft palate, base of uvula; Class IV: hard palate only.

- Investigate the posterior pharynx (modified Mallampati Classification) by having the sitting patient fully extend his neck, maximally open his mouth, and stick out his tongue with or without phonation. Figure 2.1 shows how we classify the visible structures.
- Determine the ability to move lower in front of the upper incisors, which is a good sign.
- Evaluate neck mobility: full extension through full flexion should exceed 90°. Patients who require further evaluation include:
  (i) those with rheumatoid arthritis and/or Down's syndrome: the transverse ligament that secures the odontoid can become lax, introducing the potential for cervical cord trauma with direct laryngoscopy;
  (ii) trauma patients who may have damaged their cervical spine (Table 2.1).
- Finally, patients with a history of difficult intubation and any obvious airway pathology (vocal cord tumor, neck radiation scar, congenital malformation, etc.)

Fig. 2.2 Mask–ventilation technique.

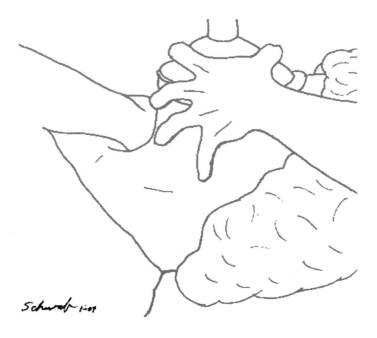

Fig. 2.2 Mask–ventilation technique.

should be further investigated. Patients with a history of snoring and/or morbid obesity also cause us concern.

See http://www.anest.ufl.edu/EA for a thorough review of airway evaluation.

Airway management techniques

Mask–ventilation

Simple as it seems, the ability to mask–ventilate a patient is *the* essential airway management technique that needs to be practised and learned by every health-care provider. Most important is the patient's head position: Do not let the patient's neck flex and thus potentially occlude the airway, which makes mask–ventilation difficult to impossible. Proper mask technique includes the following:

  (i) Select an appropriate size mask to fit over the patient's nose and mouth and provide an airtight seal without pressure on the eyes.

 (ii) Place the head in sniffing position (occiput elevated, neck extended) or directly supine, with the neck neutral to slightly extended.

(iii) Positioning yourself at the patient's head, apply the mask to the face with a pincer grip by thumb and index finger of the left hand. Place the third finger on the mentum and pull the chin upward. The fourth finger remains on the mandible so as not to compress the soft tissue, with the pinkie at the angle of the mandible where the jaw can be pushed forward to open the posterior pharynx (a painful maneuver in an awake patient!) (Fig. 2.2).

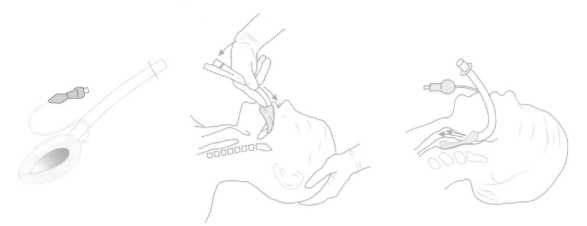

Fig. 2.3 Laryngeal mask airway. We advance the LMA along the roof of the mouth of the anesthetized patient, until it seats at the esophageal inlet. We inflate the cuff, which causes the LMA to rebound slightly. Finally, we confirm placement by the presence of end-tidal CO_2 on the capnograph. LMA = laryngeal mask airway.

(iv) Then ventilate the patient's lungs with a self-inflating bag, Mapleson or anesthesia machine circle system. Keep inflation pressures to the minimum required to ventilate the lungs, in an effort to prevent inflation of the stomach.

What to do when mask–ventilation proves to be difficult:

- Reposition. Make sure the mandible is being pulled anteriorly.
- Add a second person to try two-handed mask–ventilation. Use both hands to hold the mask and pull the jaw anteriorly. The other person compresses the breathing bag.
- Use an oral or nasal airway to establish a pathway past the pharyngeal tissue and tongue. This is not advisable in the awake patient (he would retch) nor under light anesthesia (he might develop a tight laryngospasm, which would make matters worse). A nasal trumpet can be inserted after lubrication with a local anesthetic jelly, even if the patient is awake.
- If the patient has a beard, try placing an occlusive dressing (with a hole for the mouth) over the beard, or apply Vaseline to the mask.
- The edentulous patient usually does better with his false teeth in place. If the patient is comatose, an oral airway may help, or stuff the cheeks with gauze to provide enough shape for the mask to seal properly. Just be sure to remove all material from the mouth when the patient is ready to resume spontaneous breathing – material left behind has been aspirated and has caused acute airway obstruction and death!

Laryngeal mask airway

Developed in the 1980s, the laryngeal mask airway (LMA; Fig. 2.3) has supplanted tracheal intubation for many general anesthetics. The device is basically the progeny of a facemask mated with an endotracheal tube, allowing positioning of the mask just above the glottic opening. While we have available a version intended to protect the airway from gastric aspiration (LMA Proseal®), none can guarantee it. The major advantages of the LMA over tracheal intubation are the lower level of skill required for placement, decreased airway trauma (especially of the vocal cords), and reduced stimulation such that lightly anesthetized, spontaneously breathing patients can tolerate the device. Also, the properly positioned LMA places the laryngeal inlet in clear view for a fiberoptic scope, making tracheal intubation through the device a popular technique in the management of the difficult airway.

To place the LMA, we induce anesthesia without paralysis, then

(i) place the patient's head in the sniffing position;

(ii) stabilize the occiput and slightly extend the neck with the right hand, allowing the jaw to fall open;

(iii) press the deflated LMA against the hard palate with the gloved index finger, and gently advance it until encountering the resistance of the upper esophageal sphincter.

There are many variations to this technique, including the popular initial insertion upside-down, then rotation in the posterior pharynx (not recommended by the manufacturer). When difficulty arises, try moving to the front of the patient, placing the right hand on the top of the LMA and using the index finger to coax the tip of the LMA down toward the laryngeal inlet. Any restriction to the mouth opening makes that impossible. When correctly positioned, the cuff comes to sit at the base of the hypopharynx. The vocal cords (and many times the esophagus) will come into view within the LMA bowl. Thus, this airway does not protect against aspiration. While it can be used during controlled ventilation, we risk gastric distension if inflation pressure exceeds 20 cm H_2O.

We remove the LMA from the awake patient after suctioning above the cuff and then deflating it. Because the LMA is less stimulating than an endotracheal tube, and unlikely to produce laryngospasm upon its removal, in the spontaneously breathing patient the LMA can be removed in the PACU by nursing staff, thereby reducing anesthetic wake-up time in the OR and improving OR throughput.

Endotracheal intubation

Oral intubation by direct laryngoscopy

We prefer to intubate the trachea when we need to have more control of the patient's airway, ventilate his lungs, and protect against aspiration of gastric contents. The use of a cuffed tracheal tube (Fig. 2.4) reduces the risk of aspiration in the adult.[1] Our first step is to confirm all necessary equipment is at hand:

• a properly checked anesthesia machine, or a self-inflating bag or Mapleson system with source of compressed oxygen, and a tight fitting mask;

• endotracheal tubes (ETT) of appropriate sizes (see Table 2.2). Generally we like to have an extra tube $1/2$ size smaller than that anticipated . . . just in case;

• a stylet that fits in the ETT – sometimes required to stiffen and shape the tube;

Table 2.2. Endotracheal tube sizes and approximate depths

Group	ETT size (mm ID)	ETT depth (cm from alveolar ridge)
Children	(4 + age)/4	(12 + age)/2
Adult women	7.0–8.0	20–22 cm
Pregnant women	6.5–7.5	20–22 cm
Adult men	8.0–9.0	22–24 cm

ETT = endotracheal tube.

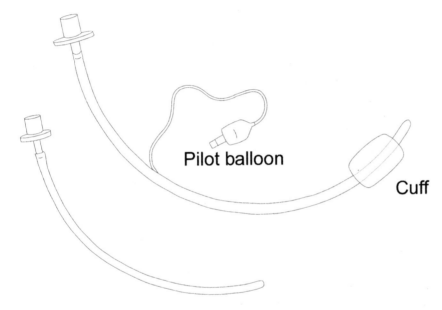

Pilot balloon

Cuff

Fig. 2.4 Adult and pediatric endotracheal tubes. Note there is no cuff on the pediatric tube.

- a syringe to inflate the ETT cuff;
- an oral airway, in case intubation and mask ventilation prove to be difficult;
- laryngoscope handle and appropriate blades (Fig. 2.5), usually at least a curved (Macintosh) and straight (Miller), with confirmation that the light works!
- suction – for the inevitable oral secretions and potential regurgitation;
- induction drugs;?>
- an assistant schooled in application of cricoid pressure: manual pressure applied to the cricoid ring, compressing the esophagus against the vertebral body beneath, in hope of preventing passive regurgitation.

The smooth placement of an endotracheal tube requires skill and practice. Usually we start with denitrogenating (pre-oxygenating) the patient's lungs before rendering the patient unconscious and immobile (including paralysis of the muscles of respiration) for the intubation. If the patient cannot breathe and we are unable to ventilate his lungs, his life is in danger. Fortunately, we can usually identify

Fig. 2.5 Laryngoscope blades. The first two (Miller 0 and Miller 2) are classified as "straight" blades with which we lift the epiglottis to view the vocal cords. The last is the Macintosh 3 with handle. The tip of the blade is placed in front of the epiglottis as shown in Fig 2.6.

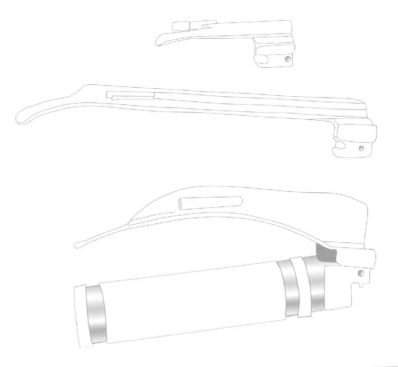

those patients in whom conventional endotracheal intubation will be difficult. It is vitally important to recognize them *before* administering medications that induce apnea.

Intubation is typically performed with direct visualization of the larynx, that is, we like to *watch* the tube pass through the vocal cords. Unfortunately, without an instrument such as the laryngoscope, no direct line of sight exists through the open mouth to the larynx. Instead, we must find a way to bring the larynx into view – enter "direct laryngoscopy." Here we position the patient's head in the "sniffing position:" flexed at the lower cervical spine and extended at the atlanto-occipital joint (see Fig. 2.6). Then we advance a laryngoscope to the level of the epiglottis and use it to pull the lower jaw and tongue up and out of the way, opening up a line of sight to the larynx (usually). The exposure of the larynx varies and has been classified by Cormack and Lehane (Fig. 2.7).

Thus, to intubate a patient with a "normal airway," first position, denitrogenate (pre-oxygenate), and induce the patient as described above, then proceed as follows:

(i) Take the laryngoscope in your left hand; the right hand is responsible for everything else.

(ii) Place the right hand on top of the patient's head and accentuate neck extension. Note that some prefer to perform a scissor-like maneuver with the right thumb and index finger to open the patient's jaw.

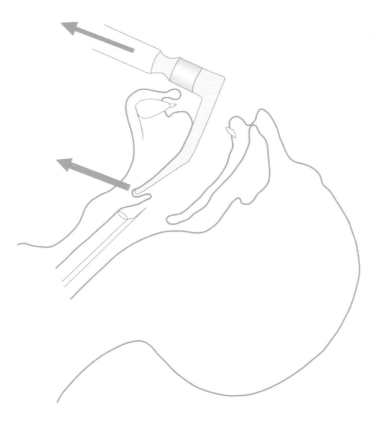

Fig. 2.6 Direct laryngoscopy. The laryngoscope is *lifted* toward the edge of the ceiling across the room, *not cranked* as that will damage the teeth and fail to provide the desired view.

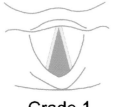

Grade 1

Grade 2

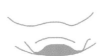

Grade 3

Grade 4

Fig. 2.7 Cormack and Lehane Classification of laryngeal view. Grade 1: full view of the glottis; Grade 2: only the posterior commissure is visible; Grade 3: only the epiglottis is seen; Grade 4: no epiglottis or glottis structure visible.

(iii) Advance the laryngoscope down the right side of the mouth to the level of the tonsillar pillars. Sweep the tongue to the left as you bring the laryngoscope to the midline.

(iv) With a straight blade, lift the epiglottis; with a curved blade, place it at the base of the epiglottis. As above, lift forward and upward (in the direction of the laryngoscope handle). Do not pry or crank with the laryngoscope! Teeth might be broken.

(v) When you can see the glottic opening clearly, grasp the endotracheal tube (hold it like a pencil – not a dagger) with the right hand (preferably without losing sight of the glottis), and advance the tip into the trachea just until the cuff disappears completely beyond the vocal cords.

(vi) Inflate the cuff only to the point of no air leakage, and *confirm tracheal position*.

This last point is *very* important. Patients do not die from esophageal intubation; they die when esophageal intubation is not recognized! You must be *absolutely* sure the tube is in the right place! A fiberoptic bronchoscope that finds the tip of the tube below the cords and above the carina would be ideal but is impractical as a clinical routine. A chest radiograph, both PA and lateral, confirming location in the trachea would also work, but is similarly impractical for OR applications. Instead, we must use clinical clues and technology.

(a) *Confirmation of exhaled CO_2 is the gold standard*, either by quantitative capnography as in the operating room, or the more mobile colorimetric sensors. Note, however, that this only guarantees ventilation of the lungs. It does not specifically identify the ETT as placed in the *trachea*. Pharyngeal position of the tube with ventilation (as with an LMA) may yield CO_2. Conversely, during cardiovascular collapse, with minimal or no pulmonary blood flow, little or no CO_2 will be returned to the lungs from the periphery, and end-tidal CO_2 might not be measurable. Place a sensor anyway because the return of detectable CO_2 will indicate effective resuscitative efforts and perfusion of the lungs.

(b) *Breath sounds* While not definitive for tracheal placement, breath sounds should be present across the chest and absent over the stomach. We can rule out endobronchial intubation when we hear good breath sounds bilaterally. Emphasis on the *bilaterally*; listening close to one side of the sternum, we often mistake breath sounds transmitted from the other side.

(c) *Condensation* While reassuring, condensation in the clear plastic ETT during exhalation is no ironclad guarantee either.

(d) *Palpation of the ETT cuff* Still not flawless, but when combined with the presence of exhaled CO_2, palpation of the cuff in the suprasternal notch (notable by the bounce felt while squeezing the pilot balloon) does confirm tracheal position.

(e) *Chest excursion* should be symmetric.

Can't intubate situations

Here the hearts (of the caregivers) begin to pound . . . when the vocal cords cannot be visualized. If this problem arises after adequate pre-oxygenation, you will have won valuable time before serious hypoxemia ensues. The first thing we try is to change the patient's position, the laryngoscope blade, and/or the laryngoscopist. If this does not help (and the patient is still apneic), then another technique must be attempted (Table 2.3).

Table 2.3. Rescue techniques when intubation fails

Non-invasive
- Continued mask ventilation
- Blind intubation (usually more successful via the nose)
- LMA; perhaps used as a conduit to intubation
- Combitube® (a blindly-placed double-lumen tube through which ventilation may be achieved regardless of its location: trachea or esophagus (provided the vocal cords are open))
- Lighted stylet (a lighted malleable stylet inside an ETT and used to identify the trachea by a pretracheal glow in the neck)
- Fiberoptic intubation (with or without LMA as a conduit)
- Intubating stylet or tube changer (more malleable than an ETT and may include a lumen through which oxygen can be insufflated into the lungs while attempting to pass the ETT)
- Retrograde intubation (a wire placed via the cricothyroid membrane is advanced into the nose or mouth, then used as a guide for intubation) – not all that non-invasive and not all that often successful.

Invasive
- Cricothyrotomy (with a needle and jet ventilation)
- Percutaneous tracheostomy (possible in a minute)
- Surgical tracheostomy (takes many minutes)

The selection of rescue technique depends on the situation, experience of the physician, availability of equipment, and whether mask–ventilation is possible. For example, "can't intubate, can't ventilate" scenarios necessitate rapid intervention, and thus, fiberoptic intubation would not be a likely choice for an inexperienced physician; placement of an LMA is much more likely to be successful. Whereas in a "can't intubate, *can* ventilate" scenario, we may be able to mask–ventilate the patient's lungs while the surgeon does a tracheostomy or wait until the patient awakens and then perform an awake fiberoptic intubation. Remember that non-depolarizing muscle relaxants cannot be reversed until the patient regains at least one twitch on the train-of-four (ulnar stimulation), which may require 30 minutes to more than an hour depending on the muscle relaxant and dose administered. For this reason, we choose short-acting drugs, e.g., succinylcholine, when we anticipate difficulties: if intubation fails, the drug effect will wear off within a few minutes, and the patient can once again breathe spontaneously.

Awake fiberoptic intubation
Sometimes an indirect visualization technique becomes necessary, either during airway rescue, or when a pre-operative examination suggests a likelihood of

Fig. 2.8 Innervation of the airway. Anterior 2/3 of the tongue – Trigeminal nerve (V); posterior 1/3 of tongue to epiglottis – Glossopharyngeal nerve (IX); epiglottis to vocal cords – Internal branch of superior laryngeal nerve (Vagus, X); trachea below vocal cords – Recurrent laryngeal nerve (Vagus, X).

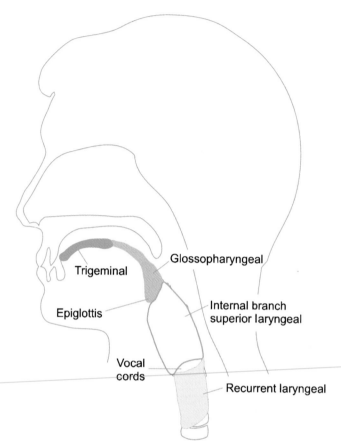

difficult intubation. In such cases, perhaps the most definitive technique is to secure the airway while the patient is still awake and breathing spontaneously. Awake fiberoptic intubation requires topical anesthesia for the patient's comfort, as well as to blunt the gag reflex that would prevent successful intubation of the trachea. All too frequently, secretions will smear the optics of the scope: an anti-sialogogue can be helpful.

Several nerves are involved in the sensation of the upper airway (Fig. 2.8). It is not much of a mnemonic, but try to remember a variant to TGIF (Thank God it's Friday) namely **TGIR**: "Thank God it's recurrent." It's lame, but perhaps just lame enough to be memorable! All but the first of these make up the gag reflex.

We anesthetize the posterior tongue and oro/nasopharynx by either spraying 4% lidocaine or having the patient gargle viscous lidocaine. Glossopharyngeal blocks also work well. We block the superior laryngeal nerves by injecting 1% lidocaine close to where the nerves penetrate the thyrohyoid membrane (Fig. 2.9). The transtracheal block is accomplished by injecting 2–4% lidocaine directly into the tracheal lumen through the cricothyroid membrane (after confirming needle

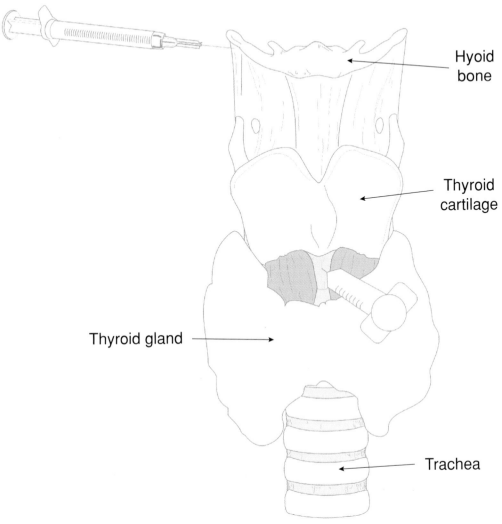

Hyoid
bone

Thyroid
cartilage

Thyroid gland

Trachea

Fig. 2.9 Airway blocks for awake
fiberoptic intubation. Location
for superior laryngeal nerve
block (top left) and transtracheal
(center) injection of local
anesthetics.

location by easily aspirating air). Be sure to point the needle toward the carina. You are very close to the vocal cords, which you do not want to damage with a needle pointed cephalad!

This technique is better tolerated with sedation, though the risk : benefit of potential airway compromise and aspiration – more likely with a numbed larynx – must always be taken into account.

Airway management plan

For many operative procedures requiring general anesthesia, any of these techniques (mask, LMA, ETT) may be appropriate, but there are times to prefer one

Table 2.4. Airway device selection

	Mask	LMA	ETT
Procedure duration	Short	Short–Medium	Any
Protects against aspiration?	No	No	Yes
Positive pressure ventilation	PIP < 20 cm H_2O	PIP < 20 cm H_2O	Any
Stimulation by device	Low	Medium	High

PIP: Peak inspiratory pressure; pressures above 20 cm H_2O may distend the stomach.

over another. We take into account the planned procedure and the patient's status (Table 2.4). An emergency laparoscopic appendectomy should probably be performed with an ETT because of the high risk of aspiration (full stomach and increased intra-abdominal pressure from laparoscopy), while a professional singer undergoing a minor elective procedure might be better served with a mask or LMA.

A word about the patient with a potentially unstable cervical spine. Many times, trauma patients arrive from the Emergency Department without a "cleared" cervical spine. Though radiographs can identify fractures and displacement, they fail to reveal torn or damaged ligaments, all pointing to instability of the cervical spine. If the patient is intoxicated or comatose and thus can give neither a useful history nor report cervical pain, we are in a quandary: the trauma patient's full stomach suggests the need for rapid sequence intubation to minimize the risk of aspiration, while direct laryngoscopy may traumatize the spinal cord. The options become these:

(i) *An airway technique* One that does not require neck movement, such as intubating through an LMA, using a lighted stylet, or retrograde intubation. In skilled hands, these techniques may be performed with relative speed. A lengthy process increases the likelihood of aspiration.

(ii) *Awake fiberoptic intubation* May be difficult in an intoxicated, uncooperative patient, and may take too long in the patient with multiple traumatic injuries.

(iii) *Blind nasal intubation* Again, skilled hands dramatically increase the likelihood of success, but this technique is contra-indicated in the presence of a base-of-skull fracture, e.g., with "raccoon eyes" or with CSF dripping from the nose, as the endotracheal tube can enter the brain.

(iv) *Direct laryngoscopy with in-line stabilization* A second person stabilizes the neck (without pulling on the head) in an effort to minimize neck extension. While probably inadequate in the patient with known cervical spine injury, this technique might be used for the patient with a low likelihood of trauma whose "clearance" was limited only by intoxication.

(v) *Awake tracheostomy* Far more invasive than the other techniques, we reserve this primarily for patients with upper airway trauma that will prevent other intubation techniques.

Regardless of the technique selected, the physician administering any general anesthetic must be prepared for a failure of that plan and ready to institute an alternative airway management technique. Finally, extra pairs of skilled hands are always useful. Call for help *early* when things are not going as planned!

NOTE

1. Cuffed ETTs are not used in children less than about 8 years of age because the cuff rests near the cricoid ring, the narrowest part of the child's airway, and may cause laryngeal edema and possibly obstruction upon extubation. In fact, we want a leak around a child's ETT at about 20 cm H_2O airway pressure.

3

Vascular access and fluid management

We tend to forget that we humans (and many of our animal relatives) are mostly water. When we think about it, we must marvel how the body stores the bulk of this water in cells and the interstitial, extracellular fluid, where much of the water is tied up in gel. Suspended in this interstitial lake is the vascular compartment, comparatively puny in volume but most important because of its rapid transport of fluids, nutrients, and waste throughout the system, and its continuous and efficient exchange of water with the interstitial compartment (Fig. 3.1). Clinically, we can see dehydration in sunken eyeballs, wrinkling skin and dry lips, or the excess of fluids in edema and swollen eyes; we can even hear it should water collect in the alveoli.

Vascular access

During anesthesia, and whenever the oral route is unavailable, we give fluids parenterally. As long as we need to give only physiologic solutions, we can administer them subcutaneously; however, the uptake and distribution of such a depot of fluids takes time. Much preferred and much faster is the intravenous route. Thus, vascular access assumes a critically important role in the peri-operative care of patients. The vascular bed also offers an ideal route for many drugs that need to be distributed throughout the body. Finally, intravascular pressures provide information on cardiovascular function. Thus, vascular access has become a skill, and fluid management a science, mastered by anesthesiologists.

Our skin is a wonderful organ. It wraps us securely into an elastic, fairly tough, self-repairing, protective envelope. When we break this envelope, we expose the patient to considerable risks. In addition to hazards associated with the actual placement of needles and catheters, infectious complications contribute significantly to morbidity and mortality of the hospitalized patient, particularly in the intensive care unit where we frequently employ central venous access. Infectious complications include local site infection, catheter-related bloodstream

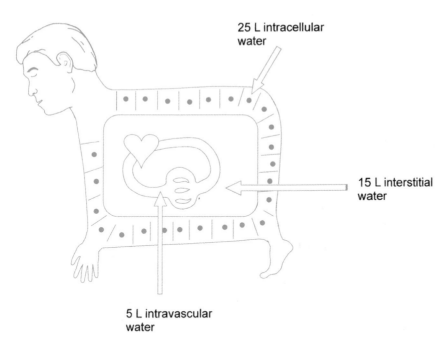

25 L intracellular water

15 L interstitial water

5 L intravascular water

Fig. 3.1 An uncharitable view (not to scale) of a 70 kg man as a tub filled with water (amounting to 60% of his body weight). This water is tucked away in cells (~65%), caught in the extracellular (interstitial) space (~25%) and circulating in the intravascular compartment (~10%).

infections, septic thrombophlebitis, endocarditis, and other metastatic infections such as osteomyelitis and abscesses of lung or brain.

Peripheral venous cannulation

Let's go through the steps involved:

(i) *Explain the need* for vascular access and obtain consent from the patient. Parents can be of great help in preparing a child for an i.v.

(ii) *Topicalize* If there is sufficient time (30–45 minutes), a topical anesthetic such as EMLA (eutectic mixture of local anesthetics) can be applied to the intended site. In our practice, this is only worthwhile for small children.

(iii) *Acquire equipment (Table 3.1)* We usually select the largest catheter appropriate for the selected vein.

(iv) *Don clean gloves* They need not be sterile. From now on, you are dealing with the patient's blood, and you should expose neither yourself nor the patient to the possibility of infection.

(v) *Select the site* This involves more than just looking for the most visible vein. We often use the back of the hand because veins are both visible and easy to immobilize. Things to consider: use the non-dominant hand, avoid "creases" where kinking is likely, e.g., wrist, seek a relatively straight vein without venous valves that may hinder its cannulation; inserting at a venous fork is helpful

Table 3.1. Equipment for peripheral intravenous access

Tourniquet
Gloves (that fit – you, not the patient)
Site prep, e.g., chlorhexidine
Local anesthetic (1% lidocaine plain ~0.5 ml and 25–27 g needle)
i.v. catheter (? gauge, ? length) × 2 in case of a miss
4×4 sponge (to clean up afterward)
Clear occlusive dressing
Pre-torn tape
i.v. fluids, primed and free of bubbles

as the vein tends to be better stabilized. Finally, we do not cannulate an arm that has been the target of an arteriovenous shunt (as for dialysis) or a lymph node dissection (as in a mastectomy).

(vi) *Apply a tourniquet* Should be tight enough to obstruct venous return without restricting arterial flow. Do not actually tie a knot, just fold one side under the other.

(vii) *Prepare the site* We prefer to use a bactericidal agent such as chlorhexidine; next best would be an iodine-containing solution, e.g., betadine, which must be allowed to dry and should not be wiped off with alcohol. Finally, a patient allergic to both of the above should be washed with alcohol alone.

(viii) *Inject local anesthetic* Awake patients benefit greatly if we take the time to first anesthetize their skin. It requires only a tiny volume (~0.1 mL) of local anesthetic injected immediately adjacent to (not over) the vein, minimizing the risk of obscuring visibility of the vein. While injection of lidocaine burns, we can reduce the discomfort by:

- Counter-irritation – with a free finger, scratch the patient's skin near the injection site, this "confuses" the nerve endings and reduces pain.
- Alkalinize the lidocaine – add 1 mL bicarbonate (8.4%) to every 10 mL lidocaine.

Some argue that using local anesthesia insures two sticks instead of one, and that a "needle is a needle." We beg to differ: first, the local should be administered with a 25–27 g needle, which is barely felt by most patients; second, the i.v. does not always go in on the first try; and third, the pain of the needle without local is worse than the local anesthetic injection (personal experience).

(ix) *Stabilize the vein* with traction below the puncture site.

(x) *Puncture the skin* at a 30–45-degree angle (through the local anesthetic wheal!).

(xi) *Proceed into the vein* either directly from above or from the side; make sure you can see the plastic hub of the needle to observe the return of blood.

(xii) *Advance catheter* When you see a flash of blood, reduce your angle and advance a tiny amount (literally 1–2 mm), then feed the catheter off the needle. Fully advance the catheter before pulling out the needle. You cannot thread the flexible catheter without the stiff needle as a stylet, and the needle cannot be reinserted as the catheter may be punctured.

(xiii) *Remove the tourniquet* (facilitated by proper placement in the first place).

(xiv) *Apply gentle pressure* over the tip of the catheter to prevent bleeding back.

(xv) *Remove the needle* and dispose in a "Sharps" container.

(xvi) *Connect i.v. fluid* administration set and open to observe free flow, then slow down the administration as indicated by the patient's condition.

(xvii) *Observe the i.v. site* to confirm intravascular and not interstitial placement (not foolproof but helpful).

(xviii) *Secure the i.v.* With due respect to those who consider this an art form, find a method that allows visibility of the entry site (to observe for infection) and the area over the tip of the catheter (to detect infiltration). Secure the i.v. so that motion will not dislodge it. A loop in the tubing prevents a small amount of traction from pulling directly on the catheter.

The fluid administered depends on the goal for the infusion. In general, fluids should be administered through a programmable pump with adequate safety measures. That said, in anesthesia we usually control the rate of fluid administration through the i.v. tubing's roller clamp. In this case, *do not hang more fluid than you want the patient to receive*. For an infant, do not hang a liter bag without a buretrol (a 150–200 mL reservoir attached between the i.v. fluid bag and the catheter). If the roller clamp is inadvertently left open, the patient will not be fluid overloaded.

When we recognize the potential need for rapid fluid administration (read: major blood letting), we plan our intravenous access accordingly. The maximum attainable flow rate depends on the resistance of the system, including the length and diameter of everything from the tubing to the vein itself. So, remove any small diameter connectors and select a shorter, larger catheter (at least an 18 g in an adult).[1] Selecting a large vein for rapid flow is obvious, but the effect of cold fluids may be underestimated. Finally, two medium bore i.v.s accommodate more fluid than a single large bore.

Central venous catheterization

The complication rate of central venous catheterization (Table 3.2) is much higher than for peripheral i.v.s, thus the first question should be whether central venous cannulation is truly necessary (Table 3.3). When placed emergently, for instance in a trauma patient, these catheters should be replaced within 48 hours to reduce the risk of infection.

Table 3.2. Complications of central venous catheterization and how to prevent them

One or the other complication occurs in more than 15% of patients undergoing central venous catheterization.

Infectious complications 5–26%:
- Use antimicrobial impregnated catheters.
- Avoid the femoral route; subclavian (SC) might be better than Internal jugular vein (IJ).
- Employ sterile technique (including mask, cap, gown, gloves, drape, etc.).
- Avoid antibiotic ointment at insertion site (this encourages resistant organisms and fungi).
- Disinfect catheter hubs when injecting or attaching tubing.
- Minimize duration of catheterization.

Mechanical complications 5–19%: the most common are arterial puncture (Femoral>IJ>SC), hematoma and pneumothorax (SC>IJ).

- Optimize likelihood of success including proper positioning of the patient.
- Use ultrasound guidance during IJ catheterization – this speeds the process, improves the success rate, and reduces the risk of hitting the carotid artery.
- Use a "finder needle" if ultrasound guidance is unavailable – this smaller gauge needle makes a much smaller hole if it ends up in the wrong place. The introducer needle is then advanced along the finder needle into the vein.

Thrombotic complications 2–26%: most common with femoral site, probably least common for SC.

Table 3.3. Indications for central venous catheterization

- Need (anticipated or actual) to infuse fluids at a great rate
- Administration of agents that require a central route (some vasoactive drugs, hyperalimentation, high concentrations of electrolytes)
- Need to transduce central pressures (pulmonary artery and occlusion pressures as well as cardiac output may be available with a pulmonary artery catheter)
- Stable venous access in patients without other accessible sites, e.g., morbid obesity

The next question deals with access site. The three most common insertion sites are as follows:

- *Femoral* Probably technically the easiest (remember, from lateral to medial, NAVEL – nerve, artery, vein, empty space, lymphatics) and quickest, with the lowest rate of serious complications (though highest rate of minor complications), but these catheters are more difficult to keep clean and therefore more likely to be a source of infection.
- *Subclavian (SC)* Once placed, this catheter location is probably the most comfortable for the patient. Unfortunately, it carries a significant risk of pneumothorax (up to 3%), and the procedure can be very difficult when landmarks are obscured, as in obesity.

Table 3.4. Types of central venous catheters

- Antimicrobial-impregnated – this is important! It reduces catheter-related bloodstream infections.
- Single vs multilumen – depends on the intended use. If multiple drugs need be infused simultaneously, a multilumen catheter should be selected.
- Pulmonary artery (PA) catheter – if we want pulmonary artery or occlusion pressures, or cardiac output determination, a PA catheter (also known as a Swan–Ganz catheter) will do the trick. There are many types of these with variable capabilities (thermodilution cardiac output, continuous cardiac output, pacing port, etc.), make sure you check carefully before opening the (expensive) package.

- *Internal jugular (IJ)* Anesthesiologists favor this location because of accessibility (we're already at the head of the patient) and the low risk of pneumothorax. Incidentally, we prefer the right IJ over the left due to the "straightness" of the route to the heart and because we need not worry about the left-sided thoracic duct.

In addition to selecting a catheter size appropriate to the patient and indication, there are other features to consider (Table 3.4).

Because the majority of catheters in anesthesia are placed in the IJ location in an anesthetized patient, we will describe this technique. In an awake patient, we would add sedation, continual reassurance, and local anesthesia.

IJ catheter placement technique
Once we have confirmed the need for central venous catheterization, obtained the patient's consent, and collected all equipment, we work as follows:

(i) Optimally position the patient: Trendelenburg's position[2] (head-down, to increase the size of the vein and prevent air embolism), with the head turned about 45 degrees to the opposite side.

(ii) Prepare: gown, sterile gloves, cap, mask, with catheter tray open and in easy reach.

(iii) Prepare the site: we prefer chlorhexidine, but an iodine solution that has dried can be substituted depending on the patient's allergies.

(iv) Identify the insertion point: while there are many possible sites along the vessel, we advocate a mid to high approach, minimizing the possibility of pneumothorax. One technique: place the third finger of the left hand in the sternal notch, the thumb on the mastoid process, and then bisect the line with the index finger, adjusting to palpate the carotid at this level. Do not try to push the carotid out of the way, as both vessels lie in the same sheath. If the external jugular vein crosses at this location, move above or below it.

(v) Using a finder needle (22–23 g) attached to a syringe, begin about 1 cm lateral to the carotid pulse, aiming toward the ipsilateral nipple. Advance the needle through the skin, then gently aspirate on the plunger as you slowly advance the needle. In the average patient, the IJ should be no more than about 1.5 cm deep. If blood is not aspirated, slowly withdraw the needle and adjust the angle slightly. First check that the vein does not lie more lateral, then cautiously check more medially and caudally.

(vi) When blood is aspirated, carefully transfer the finder needle/syringe to the left hand. With the right hand, carefully advance the introducer needle along the finder needle and into the vessel until blood is easily aspirated.

(vii) Remove the finder needle and the syringe from the introducer needle, and confirm intravenous location (see below). Keep your thumb (in a sterile glove!) over the hub of the needle when there is nothing attached to minimize blood loss and avoid a potentially catastrophic air embolism if the central venous pressure is low, or should the patient suddenly decrease it by taking a gasping breath.

(viii) Advance the wire through the needle. Here, we must monitor ECG to detect the common extra systoles. Should there be a sustained run of ventricular tachycardia, withdraw the wire a few centimeters.

(ix) Remove the needle and advance the catheter over the wire to the desired depth (sometimes there will be a dilator step in-between). Make sure to hold the wire while advancing or removing equipment over it, so as not to remove it, or (worse yet) fully insert it into the patient.

(x) Remove the wire, cap off the ports, aspirate and flush each, suture the catheter in place, and dress with a clear occlusive dressing.

(xi) Obtain a chest radiograph to confirm the catheter tip position. The optimal location for a catheter placed via the IJ or SC route is just above the right atrium, where it will not perforate atrial tissue. An X-ray can also rule out pneumothorax and can suggest an extravascular location of the catheter.

Confirmation of intravenous location

Several techniques can help to confirm that the needle is not in an artery – usually the carotid. While pulsatility and a bright red color are good hints, they are not foolproof.

- If ultrasound guidance was used to place the catheter (as is routine at our institution), use it to confirm position as well.
- Attach a length of sterile clear tubing to the needle hub and lower the end, allowing it to fill several centimeters with blood, then raise above the patient's heart level. A rising column of pulsating blood confirms arterial location, while a column that reflects the central venous pressure is a more welcome finding.

Pulmonary artery catheterization

In addition to the risks of central venous catheterization listed above, pulmonary artery (PA) catheterization has caused catastrophic pulmonary artery rupture and

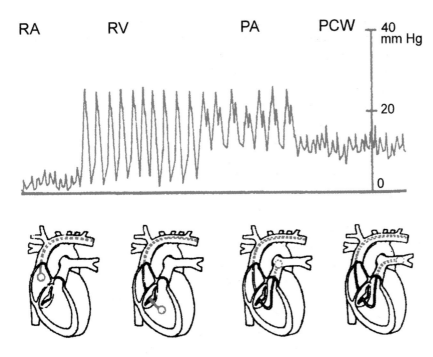

Fig. 3.2 Pressure tracings during placement of a pulmonary artery catheter. RA = right atrium; RV = right ventricle; PA = pulmonary artery; PCW = pulmonary capillary wedge. (Reproduced with permission from Dizon, C.T. and Barash, P.G. The value of monitoring pulmonary artery pressure in clinical practice. *Conn. Med.* **41**(10):623, 1977.)

comes with the increased risk of arrhythmias, complete heart block (particularly if the patient has a pre-existing left bundle branch block), pulmonary embolism, and cardiac valve damage. Thus, this invasive technique requires rigorous justification. Do you really need to have PA pressure, PA occlusion pressure (PAOP, also known as pulmonary capillary wedge pressure, PCWP), or cardiac output? And how will it affect your management?

After placing an introducer (a special large-bore central venous catheter) via the central venous access technique above, a PAC is sterilely inserted through the introducer.

(i) Prepare the catheter: flush and cap the PAC ports. Test the balloon for symmetric inflation and passive deflation on release of the syringe pressure. Connect the *PA distal* port to a pressure transducer with the monitor in view. Cover the catheter with the clear plastic sheath[3] that maintains internal sterility for subsequent manipulation of catheter depth.

(ii) Advance the catheter through the introducer to 20 cm and confirm the CVP waveform on the monitor (see below). Instruct an assistant to inflate the balloon.

(iii) Advance the catheter while keeping track of its depth as well as the waveform transduced from its tip (Fig. 3.2). The RV tracing should appear before the catheter has been advanced about 30 cm, and the PAOP before 50 cm. If they do not, deflate the balloon, pull back the catheter 10 cm or so, reinflate the

Table 3.5. Blood volume estimates

Population	Blood volume (ml/kg body weight)
Premature neonates	95
Infants	80
Adult men	70
Adult women	60

balloon and try again. Over-insertion can result in a knot, necessitating a vascular procedure to remove the catheter.

(iv) Once the PAOP tracing is obtained, deflate the balloon and confirm reappearance of the PA trace. If this does not occur, you must withdraw the catheter a few centimeters. Continue manipulation until the PA trace with the balloon deflated becomes the PAOP (or wedge) trace on inflation. Always inflate the balloon to just barely occlude the PA pressure in order to avoid rupturing the vessel. And remember . . . *balloon up on catheter advancement, balloon down on withdrawal.*

(v) Aspirate to confirm intravascular location, and flush all ports. Obtain a chest radiograph to confirm proper location (within the mediastinal shadow).

Fluid management

As mentioned at the start of this chapter, we are mostly water, actually salt water with some other chemicals thrown in for good measure. The intravascular compartment, replete with cells and proteins, differs from the rest of the body. In fact the blood volume also differs with age and sex (Table 3.5). We may lose fluid in a number of ways, from the obvious – hemorrhage, urine, vomiting – to the less obvious – sweat, evaporation from exposed viscera or trachea, transudation between compartments. While fluid escapes from anywhere, replacement occurs only through the intravascular compartment.

Fluid types

Many types of fluids are available for intravascular administration (Table 3.6).
- *Crystalloid*
  - *Hypotonic solutions* With an osmolality less than that of serum (285–295 mOsm/kg), these are rarely used in anesthesia (except pediatrics), because very little of the infused fluid remains intravascularly ($<10\%$ of D_5W), electrolytes are diluted, and cells swell.

Table 3.6. Composition of common intravenous fluids

	Na^+ (mEq/L)	Cl^- (mEq/L)	K^+ (mEq/L)	Ca^{2+} (mEq/L)	Other	Approximate pH	Calculated mOsm/L
D_5W					Dextrose 5 g/L	5.0	253
Normal saline	154	154				4.2	308
Ringer's lactate	130	109	4.0	3.0	Lactate 28 mEq/L	6.5	273
Hespan	154	154			Hydroxyethyl starch, 6 g/dL	5.5	310
3% NaCl	513	513				5.0	1027
In normal serum	136–145	98–106	3.5–5.1	4.2–5.3		7.35–7.45	275–295*

* Serum osmolarity is estimated as $2 \times [Na^+] + glucose/18 + BUN/2.8$.

- *Isotonic solutions* Preferred, though still only about 25% of the infused volume remains intravascularly, with the rest seeping into the interstitial space; representatives include 0.9% sodium chloride (also known as normal saline) and lactated Ringer's (which also contains potassium and calcium).
- *Hypertonic solutions* Available in solutions from 1.8% to 10% NaCl; 3% is the most common. While almost 65% of the infused volume remains intravascularly, these solutions may cause cellular dehydration, hypernatremia, and hyperchloremic metabolic acidosis.
- *Colloid* Containing large molecules, these solutions tend to remain intravascularly (assuming capillary integrity).
  - *Hespan® (hetastarch, hydroxyethyl starch)* Associated with coagulation abnormalities with infusions of >1 L.
  - *Pentastarch* Hetastarch's younger brother, allegedly with less effect on coagulation.
  - *Albumin* Very expensive; often refused by Jehovah's Witnesses.
- *Blood or blood components* Associated with many risks and expense (see below).
  - *Blood substitutes* We need solutions capable of carrying oxygen, without the risks and expense of blood transfusions. Unfortunately, as of this writing, these solutions – including perfluorochemical emulsions, stroma-free hemoglobin and synthetic hemoglobin – remain in clinical trials.

Fluid requirements

We calculate the intra-operative fluid requirement as follows:
  (i) *Maintenance* The 4–2–1 rule (Table 3.7) provides a guide for hourly isotonic fluid requirements.
      For a 70 kg man, this would amount to $40 + 20 + 50 = 110$ mL/h.
  (ii) *Fasting replacement* We apply the 4–2–1 rule for the duration of fasting and replace 50% over the first hour, then 25% over each of the next two hours.

Table 3.7. The 4–2–1 rule for calculation of maintenance fluid requirements

Body weight	Fluid administration
For the first 10 kg	4 mL/kg/h
For the next 10 kg	Add 2 mL/kg/h
For each kg above 20 kg	Add 1 mL/kg/h

(iii) *Insensible losses* 2 mL/kg/h.

(iv) *Urine output* Replaced mL for mL.

(v) *"Third space" losses* Transfer of fluid to this sequestered, extravascular space occurs with surgical trauma, and must be replaced with isotonic solution in the short-term: 4–8 mL/kg/h depending on the degree of surgical trauma, e.g., peripheral operation vs. open abdomen.

(vi) *Blood loss* We replace small amounts with crystalloid (3 mL per mL blood lost); in larger resuscitations, colloid and/or blood is administered 1:1 with blood loss.

Intra-operatively, we gauge fluid status by tracking vital signs, surgical progress, urine output (an inexact measure), and volume replacement. If the status is unclear, we may opt for invasive monitors such as central venous or pulmonary artery pressure monitoring (see Monitoring and Anesthesia and the cardiovascular system), or transesophageal echocardiography, which enables visualization of ventricular filling.

Blood loss

When we anticipate a large blood loss, we might calculate the "allowable blood loss" (ABL) – not the amount we "allow" the surgeon to lose, but rather the volume at which we would likely need to transfuse.

$$\text{ABL} = \frac{(Hct_{initial} - Hct_{allowed})}{(Hct_{initial} + Hct_{allowed})/2} \times EBV$$

where we use the initial and minimum acceptable hematocrits, and the estimated blood volume (Table 3.5). Unfortunately, we struggle to determine when we have reached the ABL. We report the estimated blood loss by looking at the surgical field, checking the volume in the suction canisters (subtracting any irrigation used), and examining the surgical sponges (a soaked 4×4 holds about 15 mL blood, a soaked lap sponge, 150 mL). More accurate, but generally impractical measures include weighing the sponges or washing them out and checking the color of the effluent. *In lieu* of an accurate measure, we use hemodynamic clues as well as serial hemoglobin concentrations.

This brings up the common misconception that we can assess blood loss by checking the hematocrit or hemoglobin concentration. Unless the patient has been carefully hydrated back to "euvolemia" (normal total blood volume), this is *not true*! Only if an equal volume of some other fluid is added (either from the interstitial space, or by us) does the hematocrit fall. If left to nature's device, it may take up to 2 days to reach steady state. Depending on the fluid, often much more than the actual blood loss must be given to account for the small percentage that actually remains intravascularly. The volume that escapes is not lost though; it replenishes the interstitial space that so generously donated fluid to the blood stream before treatment could be instituted. This replenishment is vital for the transport of oxygen between the blood and tissues. Massive hemorrhage and hypotension compromise oxygen delivery to tissues; to maintain cellular integrity, these cells resort to anaerobic metabolism, with a by-product of lactic acid. We often gauge our resuscitation by the severity of the lactic acidosis.

Blood replacement

As reviewed elsewhere (see Anesthesia and other systems: the blood), the trigger for red cell transfusion is based not on a single laboratory value, but rather on an assessment of the adequacy of oxygen delivery. When we deem replacement necessary – after considering the risk : benefit ratio and the wishes of the patient, e.g., Jehovah's Witness – we must decide what products to order.

Blood transfusions need to be ABO compatible. There are four major types, plus the rhesus factor (Table 3.8). In an emergency, when type-specific blood is not available, O^- ("negative") blood can serve as a "universal donor." Because only about 7% of the population has this blood type (and not all happen to be blood donors), and 90% of the population is Rh^+, it is usually safe to use O^+ blood in an emergency, at least in men. A problem arises for Rh^- women who might some day carry an Rh^+ fetus. Maternal anti-Rh antibodies will cross the placenta, causing potentially fatal erythroblastosis fetalis.

For nearly all transfusions, we administer packed cells (rather than whole blood – which enables us to collect plasma for separate infusion). For type O transfusions, this minimizes the administration of type O serum with its anti-A and anti-B antibodies. Once we have given more than four units of type O packed cells, we are obliged to continue with type O transfusions because of the administered antibody load. Lacking antibodies to A, B and Rh makes type AB^+ patients the universal recipient. A pity that they are a distinct minority (3%)!

Pre-operatively, the expected need for blood transfusions covers the spectrum from: the patient will certainly not require a transfusion (no need to determine the patient's blood type) to: we know that without several transfusions the patient

Table 3.8. Blood types and their frequencies in the population

Type	Frequency	Antibodies	PRBC	FFP, cryo, platelets
A	45%	Anti-B	A or O	A, AB
B	8%	Anti-A	B or O	B, AB
AB	4%		Any	AB
O	43%	Anti-A and anti-B	O	Any
Rh^+	90%		Any	Any
Rh^-	10%	$+/-$ Anti-Rh^+	Rh^-	Any

For platelets, as long as they are "packed" and therefore containing a low antibody titer, any type can be transfused in any patient, though we prefer to use Rh^- in women. When transfusing platelets of an incompatible blood type, the packs must be red cell free.

cannot survive (we must prepare several units of blood for this patient). To negotiate the area between these extremes, we can do the following:

(a) "Type and screen": The patient's blood is ABO and Rh typed and screened for common antibodies (indirect Coombs test). This quick and inexpensive test (if there is anything in today's hospital that can be called inexpensive) misses only about the 1% of uncommon antibodies and is therefore usually sufficient, unless the patient has had multiple transfusions in the past and has developed many unusual antibodies.

(b) "Type and crossmatch": The patient's blood is typed and the type-matched (potential) donor's cells are exposed to the patient's serum. This is more involved than type and screen, costs more money and takes more time, but readies donor blood for an immediate transfusion. We request a specific number of units to be typed and crossmatched if experience tells us to expect a large blood loss.

When we call the blood bank and ask for blood to transfuse, they always crossmatch it first, significantly delaying its arrival at the bedside. The ordering of type-specific blood is an option, though there are risks of incompatibility. Thus the time to call the blood bank is EARLY when things are not going as planned. Table 3.9 provides some basic transfusion guidelines, though we encourage you to check for updates regularly. Table 3.8 describes which products may be transfused, based on the patient's blood type.

Depending on the storage medium employed, packed red blood cells come to us with a hematocrit of 50–80%, the latter a very viscous suspension that does not infuse well. We often dilute the PRBC unit with 50–100 mL of isotonic saline (addition of hypotonic solutions will cause cell lysis, while calcium-containing fluids, e.g., Ringer's lactate, can initiate *in vitro* coagulation in contact with citrated blood). Blood is stored at 1 °C to 6 °C and should be infused through a warmer.

Table 3.9. Transfusion guidelines

Packed red blood cells (PRBC)

- Rarely transfuse if Hgb >10 g/dL; almost always if Hgb <6 g/dL
- If Hgb is 6–10 g/dL, base decision on patient's risk for complications of inadequate oxygen delivery
- Consider pre-operative autologous blood donation, cell saver (intra-operative blood recovery and re-infusion), acute normovolemic hemodilution

Platelets

- Prophylactic transfusion for surgery usually indicated if <50/μL; or <100/μL and high risk of bleeding; not indicated for states of increased destruction, e.g., ITP
- Indicated for microvascular bleeding with <50/μL; or <100/μL and risk for increased bleeding
- May be indicated despite adequate platelet count if there is known platelet dysfunction and microvascular bleeding
- Transfuse 1 u/10 kg
- 1 single donor unit $\cong$ 6 random donor units

Fresh frozen plasma (FFP)

- Urgent reversal of warfarin therapy (5–8 mL/kg)
- Correction of known coagulation factor deficiencies for which specific concentrates are unavailable
- Correction of microvascular bleeding with elevated (>1.5 times normal) PT or PTT, or when suspected factor depletion as after transfusion of more than one blood volume
- Give enough to achieve at least 30% of normal plasma factor concentration (10–15 ml/kg)
- Platelets for transfusion also contain plasma: 4–5 u platelets or 1 single-donor unit contains factors equal to about 1 u FFP

Cryoprecipitate

- Prophylactic use in perioperative or peripartum patients with congenital fibrinogen deficiencies or von Willebrand's disease unresponsive to desmopressin (DDAVP, 1-deamino-8-D-arginine vasopressin)
- Bleeding in patients with von Willebrand's disease
- Correction of microvascular bleeding in massively transfused patients with fibrinogen <80 mg/dL (normal 150–450 mg/dL)
- 1u/10 kg cryoprecipitate increases plasma fibrinogen by 50 mg/dL

Guidelines published in *Anesthesiology* 1996; **84**:732–47.

We use special infusion sets that contain a filter (170-micron) to trap any clots or other debris.

Risks

Blood transfusions are inherently dangerous (Table 3.10). In addition to the frequent non-hemolytic reactions, ABO incompatibility threatens the potential of a hemolytic reaction with hypotension, hematuria, and fever. The diagnosis can be made more readily if the patient is awake since the symptoms of nausea, vomiting, flank or back pain and dizziness frequently accompany a transfusion reaction. Therapy includes stopping the infusion immediately (we

Table 3.10. Transfusion reactions

Transfusion reaction	Incidence	Comments
Non-hemolytic reaction	1:100–5:100	Fever, chills, urticaria
Hemolytic reaction	1:25 000	Hypotension, tachycardia, hemoglobinuria, microvascular bleeding, DIC; fatal ~1:500 000
Infectious diseases	Rare (<1:100 000)	Hepatitis A,B,C; HIV
	Significant (1:2)	CMV (immunocompromised patients should receive CMV negative units)
	Unknown	West Nile and other viruses, prions
Bacterial infection	Rare	Limit by transfusing over less than 4 hours
TRALI (transfusion related acute lung injury)	1:5 000–1:10 000	Transfused serum vs. recipient white cells; Increased capillary permeability → non-cardiogenic pulmonary edema and ARDS-type picture
Other		Dilutional thrombocytopenia, citrate toxicity → hypocalcemia

These figures are frequently updated as new screening tests become available.

return both the remaining banked blood and a sample from the patient for testing), treating mild symptoms with antihistamines and acetaminophen to reduce fever, and perhaps adding corticosteroids to reduce the immune response. We worry most about the potential for shock, kidney failure, and disseminated intravascular coagulation (DIC). In this last nasty syndrome, the antigen/antibody reaction can trigger factor XII (Hageman) which kicks the kinin system into action leading to the generation of bradykinin and, through it, damage of endothelium (oozing), hypotension, and thrombosis via the release of endogenous tissue thromboplastin. Human error plays a large part in transfusion reactions, which account for more than half of transfusion-related deaths ... translation, *double check all blood (patient and donor blood types) before transfusing!*

Unfortunately, there are several types of transfusion reactions, and some can manifest even several days after the transfusion.

As we are largely water, maintenance of the patient's fluid status represents one of anesthesiology's greatest challenges. Using vigilance, anticipation, appropriate monitors, and vascular access, we manage fluids, blood, and blood products to maintain stability and perfusion of vital organs.

NOTES

1. The traditional units of measure can be very confusing. Larger catheters are measured in "French" (or Charrière), with 3 Fr to the mm. In contrast "gauge," an inverse unit of

measure, defines needles and intravenous catheters. Each successive increase in "gauge" represents a decrease in diameter of about 10%. Thus a 21 g i.v. catheter is only about 50% the size of a 16 g.

2. Named for Friedrich Trendelenburg (the emphasis is actually on the "Trend," not the "del," as still pronounced by his family) – 1844–1924; his original description was a 45° head-down angle (we do much less) with the legs and feet hanging off the bed (actually draped over the shoulders of an assistant).

3. Locally called a Swandom.

4

Regional anesthesia

We can imagine future clinicians to prescribe treatments that would exclusively affect a single cell type or a specific organ without spillover effects. That type of explicit therapy would be the opposite to general anesthesia, the name of which implies generalized effects of the anesthetic drugs. Indeed, anesthetics delivered via the lungs or by intravenous injection flood all organs in the body, causing numerous undesired effects. How much better to pinpoint the effect with regional anesthesia. Here, we deliver the drug directly to the nervous tissue where we hope to cause a specific effect. We are closer to the ideal but not quite in heaven because we still have to contend with side effects that arise when the anesthetic drug appears in the circulation. We also lack the specificity of drugs that would block only one type of fiber and spare all others. Nevertheless, regional anesthesia provides a tool that can be used to great advantage for many patients.

Four distinct processes lead to the sensation of pain (Fig. 4.1):

(i) *Transduction* Noxious stimulation of a peripheral receptor releases local inflammatory mediators that cause changes in the activity and sensitivity of sensory neurons. *Pre-incisional* infiltration of local anesthetics effectively blocks transduction.

(ii) *Transmission* Once the noxious stimulus has been transduced, the impulses travel via A-delta and C fibers to the dorsal horn of the spinal column where they synapse. The dorsal horn cells may be subject to "wind-up" or enhanced excitability and sensitization. Transmission can be blocked with regional anesthesia.

(iii) *Perception* Afferent fibers from the dorsal horn travel to higher CNS centers, mostly via the spinothalamic tracts. Activation of the reticular formation probably increases arousal and contributes the emotional component of pain. Central-acting agents such as opioids alter perception.

(iv) *Modulation* Efferent pathways including inhibitory neurotransmitters modify the afferent nociceptive information.

The complexity of pain perception goes beyond this quick anatomic/physiologic summary. Strong emotional stimuli and distraction can completely block pain perception, as is often true for injuries sustained in battle (or when being eaten

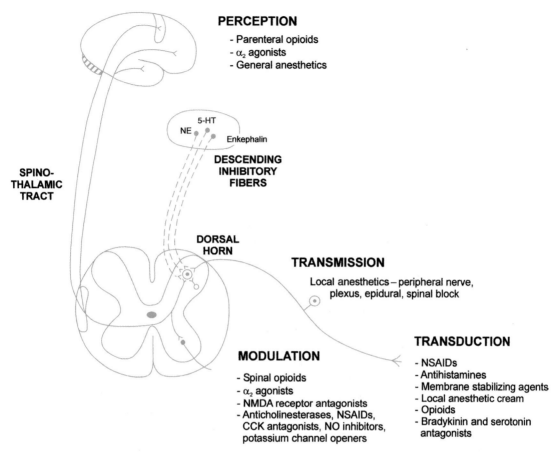

PERCEPTION
- Parenteral opioids
- α_2 agonists
- General anesthetics

5-HT
NE
Enkephalin

DESCENDING INHIBITORY FIBERS

SPINO-THALAMIC TRACT

DORSAL HORN

TRANSMISSION

Local anesthetics – peripheral nerve, plexus, epidural, spinal block

MODULATION
- Spinal opioids
- α_2 agonists
- NMDA receptor antagonists
- Anticholinesterases, NSAIDs, CCK antagonists, NO inhibitors, potassium channel openers

TRANSDUCTION
- NSAIDs
- Antihistamines
- Membrane stabilizing agents
- Local anesthetic cream
- Opioids
- Bradykinin and serotonin antagonists

Fig. 4.1 Pain processes. See text for explanation. NE = norepinephrine; 5-HT = serotonin; NMDA = N-methyl-D-aspartate; NSAID = non-steroidal anti-inflammatory; CCK = cholecysto-kinin; NO = nitric oxide. (Reproduced with permission from Kelly, D. J. *et al.* Preemptive analgesia I: physiological pathways and pharmacological modalities. *Can. J. Anesth.* **48**(10): 1001, 2001.)

by a lion). Thus, in addition to the described processes of getting the signal from injured tissue to the brain, psychological factors modulate the pain experience.

While we can interfere with the impulses traveling up the nervous pathways at any stage, mounting evidence suggests that multi-modal and pre-emptive (before incision) therapy can both improve immediate post-operative pain control and reduce the risk of a subsequent chronic pain syndrome.

Transduction of superficial noxious stimuli can be inhibited with pre-incisional local infiltration. As the name implies, regional anesthesia involves anesthetizing a specific portion of the body, thereby preventing transmission. Because pain sensation travels via nerves (A-delta and C fibers to be specific) from the site of the injury to the spinal cord (dorsal columns) and then up to the brain, the nerve impulse can be interrupted at numerous sites. Consider an operation on the big toe. Local anesthetic infiltration suffices for only the most superficial of procedures. For anything deeper, we make use of our knowledge of the area's innervation and the anatomic course of the nerves through the body. Sensory impulses can be interrupted in several locations including the ankle, popliteal fossa, sciatic notch, or at the spinal cord level. The first three would be considered peripheral nerve blocks because they block the transmission of the "pain message" before it reaches the central nervous system. We can also block the message at the level of the central nervous system with an epidural anesthetic (which could be a caudal block), or a spinal (properly called a subarachnoid) block. Together, these last approaches are called neuraxial anesthesia. And all can be effective for big toe surgery.

When used for operative anesthesia, we typically supplement a regional block with sedation; the patient need not be aware during the procedure. A balance must be struck between the patient's comfort, and the side effects of sedation, primarily respiratory depression. Also, all our sedatives, even midazolam (Versed®), linger and produce a hangover effect. Therefore, the patient will not be fully functional following the procedure, or even for the remainder of the day. Some patients do not like this feeling and would prefer the reassuring conversation of a caring anesthesiologist over drug-induced anxiolysis.

We may be tempted to choose regional anesthesia for patients with cardiovascular or pulmonary problems, arguing that a properly conducted regional technique stresses these systems less than does a general anesthetic. Be careful! If the regional block is unsuccessful, if there are complications, or if the block wears off during the operation, the patient may require emergency general anesthesia and possibly also tracheal intubation. Similarly, regional anesthesia must be used with caution in patients with a recognized "difficult airway." If we fear difficulty managing the patient's airway, we would be ill-advised to perform a regional anesthetic to "avoid the airway" without adequate preparation (additional airway equipment, etc.).

Neuraxial anesthesia

Neuraxial anesthesia involves the placement of local anesthetics and/or opioids into the intrathecal (subarachnoid) or epidural space (Fig. 4.2), either by a single injection or by a continuous infusion catheter technique. The medications act directly on the spinal cord and, for epidurals, also on the spinal roots. This results in decreased transmission of impulses through the various nerves (Table 4.1).

Some local anesthetics have differential effects on various nerve types. For most applications, we would prefer to block only the pain impulses, but no agent is quite that specific. Bupivacaine blocks sensory more than motor fibers and is the agent of choice for labor analgesia where we desire maintenance of maternal mobility ("Push! Push!").

The dermatomal level (Fig. 4.3) achieved depends on several factors (Table 4.2). Consider a Cesarean delivery, for which we require a T4 sensory level to minimize discomfort with uterine manipulation. For an epidural, we select a

Table 4.1. Classification of nerves

Class	Size	Function
Aα (myelinated)	large	Proprioception, motor
β		Touch and pressure
γ		Motor
δ	small	Temperature, sharp pain
B (myelinated)	small	Sympathetic preganglionic
C (unmyelinated)	small	Dull pain, temperature, sympathetic postganglionic

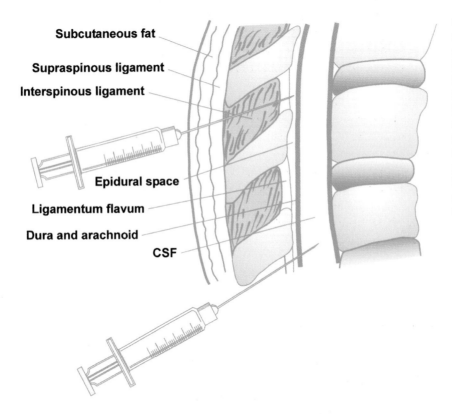

Subcutaneous fat

Supraspinous ligament

Interspinous ligament

Epidural space

Ligamentum flavum

Dura and arachnoid

CSF

Fig. 4.2 Layers of the back for neuraxial anesthesia. The upper needle demonstrates the location of the epidural space. Usually a catheter would be threaded for continuous epidural infusion of local anesthetic +/− opioids. The lower needle is in the intrathecal space, where CSF would be readily aspirated. We place intrathecal needles below the lowest extent of the spinal cord (L1-2) to minimize the risk of damage.

local anesthetic and concentration (e.g., 2% lidocaine with epinephrine), then administer ~5 mL boluses until we achieve the desired level (or we reach the maximum dose allowed). For a spinal, we administer a calculated dose and then use gravity to influence the level of the block.

Normal cerebrospinal fluid (CSF) has a specific gravity (density relative to water) of 1.0006 ± 0.0003. Any agent of a different density, injected into the CSF, will distribute according to gravity. That is, a hyperbaric agent will "sink," and hypobaric

Table 4.2. Factors determining the spread of neuraxial anesthesia

	Spinal	Epidural
Dose	Mass of drug only	Mass of drug and volume
Level of injection	Yes	Yes
Age	Yes	Yes
Patient position	Yes relative to agent baricity[a]	Minor effect
Obesity	Minor effect	Minor effect

[a] Baricity is the density (specific gravity) of the injected agent, relative to spinal fluid (see text).

Fig. 4.3 Dermatome chart. Common landmarks include the thumb at C6; nipples at T4; umbilicus at T10, iliac crest at L1, fifth toe at S1. Note that the perineum is innervated by S2-4.

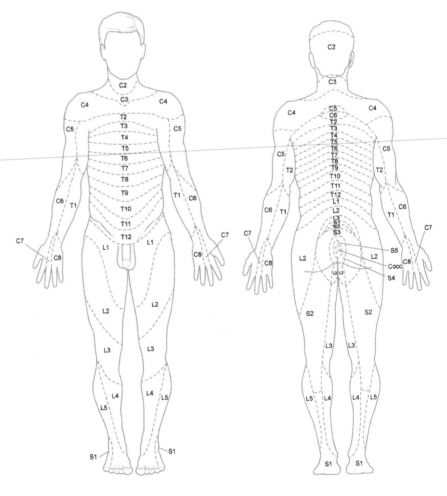

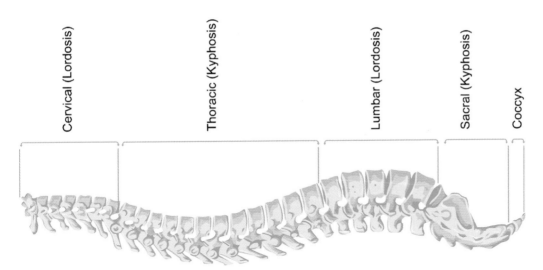

Cervical (Lordosis) · Thoracic (Kyphosis) · Lumbar (Lordosis) · Sacral (Kyphosis) · Coccyx

Fig. 4.4 Shape of the spine. Note that in the supine patient, hyperbaric intrathecal medications will "sink" to the thoracic kyphosis.

will "float." We can affect the resulting anesthetic level by tilting the patient. To achieve a T4 level for our Cesarean delivery, we inject hyperbaric local anesthetic (e.g., 12 mg of 0.75% bupivacaine with dextrose) intrathecally. When the patient assumes a supine position, the local anesthetic "sinks" to the thoracic kyphosis (Fig. 4.4). If, after a few minutes, the level of the block remains too low, we can carefully lower the patient's head; as the drug follows gravity, the level will rise.

After several minutes (the actual time depending on the agent selected), the drug will be "fixed" and no further manipulation of its level can be achieved by altering the patient's position.

Hemodynamic effects

Unfortunately, autonomic nerves (sympathetic here) are the easiest to block and cannot be independently spared. The sympathetic block extends usually at least two dermatome levels higher than the somatic sensory block. Basal sympathetic tone causes vasoconstriction peripherally, thus its elimination results in vasodilation (venous and arterial). Up to about a T4 level (nipple line), hypotension results primarily from decreased preload secondary to vasodilation proportionate to the sympathetic level (the higher the block, the more of the peripheral vasculature escapes from nervous control and is "opened"). The baroreflex response will attempt to maintain cardiac output. While its efforts to vasoconstrict the blocked area are thwarted, vasoconstriction in the unblocked area works overtime. Sympathetic stimulation reaches the heart via the "cardiac accelerators," which travel in T1–4 nerves; thus a higher block may inhibit sympathetic stimulation of the heart, resulting in bradycardia and a greater decrease of cardiac output and blood pressure.

Table 4.3. Risks and complications of neuraxial anesthesia

- Hypotension – common, often heralded by nausea (treat by increasing pre-load, cardiac output and blood pressure with volume loading; phenylephrine also finds use, especially outside the obstetric suite)
- Hypoventilation due to opioids or blockade of accessory muscles of ventilation
- Bradycardia/asystole – *rare* but requires aggressive treatment with epinephrine
- Post-dural puncture headache – probably from leaking CSF
- Local anesthetic toxicity (minimized by careful and fractionated dosing, and testing the catheter to ensure extra-vascular placement)
- Neurologic damage – epidural hematoma, cauda equina syndrome or trauma by needle – RARE
- Infection – meningitis, arachnoiditis, or epidural abscess – RARE
- Transient Radicular Irritation – usually mild buttocks/leg pain for ~1 week after spinal anesthetic – Incidence 10–20%, can be more severe with lidocaine
- Backache – usually transient
- Minor effects – urinary retention, pruritus, shivering

Pulmonary effects

If the neuraxial anesthesia level covers the thorax, intercostal muscle function will be impaired. While not a problem for most patients, those who recruit accessory muscles for normal breathing may have difficulty. Fortunately, the diaphragm receives its innervation from C2–4, and therefore the neck should never be affected by neuraxial anesthesia. If it *is*, the block is *much* too high and the patient will complain (if he still can) of dyspnea. Manual ventilation with bag and mask will be required. Often, even tracheal intubation for maintenance of the airway will become necessary. Yet, many patients become dyspneic at even a mid-thoracic level of anesthesia, and usually without any decrease in their oxyhemoglobin saturation. We attribute this to loss of chest wall proprioception, which removes a feedback loop that reassures the patient's brain that ventilation is maintained. If the patient complains of shortness of breath, first confirm that the level of anesthesia is not too high. If reassured on that point, let the patient put a hand in front of his mouth so that he can feel his exhaled breath. This may restore the feedback loop and the patient's sense of well being. If necessary, apply supplemental oxygen.

Complications

Of the potential complications to neuraxial blockade (Table 4.3), we fear formation of an epidural hematoma most. Because the spinal cord runs in the spinal canal, a closed space, anything that abnormally takes up room causes compression of other structures. Should an epidural blood vessel get nicked on insertion of a needle (common), and that vessel fail to clot normally, the resulting hematoma

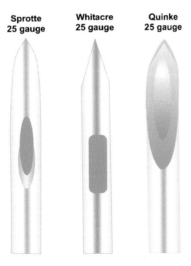

Sprotte
25 gauge

Whitacre
25 gauge

Quinke
25 gauge

Fig. 4.5 Epidural and spinal needles. The Sprotte and Whitacre are "pencil-point" needles, which are thought to *spread* the dural fibers rather than cutting them, reducing the incidence of post-dural puncture headache.

can cause increased pressure and ischemic damage to the spinal cord. For this reason, patients who are anticoagulated or thrombocytopenic are rarely considered candidates for neuraxial blocks. This risk of epidural hematoma is present both at insertion *and* removal of the catheter.

Post-dural puncture headache, another complication, deserves special mention: the patient develops pounding headaches when sitting up and finds great relief by lying down. A hole in the dura mater does not seal immediately. The size and shape of that hole has implications for the future development of a post-dural puncture (spinal) headache. We can minimize the risk of this headache by using "pencil point" needles (Fig. 4.5) in the smallest diameter practical, e.g., 25–27 g. We do not use such small diameter needles when performing a diagnostic lumbar puncture, as it would take too long to acquire fluid for laboratory studies. As you might imagine, post-dural puncture headaches are particularly bad when we inadvertently nick the dura with the large epidural needle[1] during an attempt to place an epidural catheter. This so-called "wet tap" has a high incidence of headache, particularly in the pregnant patient. Treatment includes bedrest, analgesics, intravenous caffeine, and an epidural blood patch in which the patient's own blood is sterilely injected into the epidural space, causing usually immediate relief.

Technique

Neuraxial block placement requires both skill and the patient's cooperation. Table 4.4 lists the steps for placing either a spinal or epidural anesthetic. A combined spinal–epidural (CSE) begins as an epidural, but after identification of the epidural space with the epidural needle (Fig. 4.6), a spinal needle is passed through

Table 4.4. Neuraxial blockade placement

Position patient with back flexed, sitting up or lying on the side
Identify a palpable interspace (if possible) at the desired level[a]
Put on a mask and sterile gown/gloves
Sterilely prepare and drape a wide area
Infiltrate skin and deeper planes with local anesthetic (1% lidocaine)

Spinal	Epidural
Insert guide needle, if <23 g spinal needle; smaller needles are not stiff enough to penetrate the skin.	Insert epidural needle through skin. See Fig. 4.6
Advance needle through layers: subcutaneous tissue, supraspinous ligament, interspinous ligament. If the needle is midline, there should be little pain. Redirection is required if bone is contacted.	
Increased resistance may be noted in the *ligamentum flavum*, then a "pop" as the dura is punctured. CSF returns through the needle when the stylet is removed.	Apply a glass syringe with 2–3 mL saline and a tiny air bubble. Ballotment of the syringe causes compression of the air bubble. Slowly advance the needle with continuous or intermittent ballotment until there is a "loss of resistance," where the saline is easily injected – with no compression of the bubble – into the epidural space, really a potential space that contains negative pressure when the dura is pressed upon by the needle (CAREFUL! DO NOT aspirate at this point.) Thread a catheter through the needle into the epidural space.
Apply syringe with medication, aspirate and watch for "swirl" if the densities of the CSF and local anesthetic are sufficiently different.	Attach syringe to catheter and aspirate. If you aspirate blood, the catheter tip is probably in an epidural vein. If you aspirate clear liquid, the tip may be in the subarachnoid space. But even if you cannot aspirate anything, the next step will make doubly sure.
Administer medications through the needle.	"Test dose" catheter with epinephrine-containing local anesthetic to confirm catheter is not intravascular (epinephrine-induced tachycardia) or intrathecal (rapid numbness/weakness).
Position patient for gravity-dependent spread.	Secure catheter. Position patient. Administer medications through catheter. Start with conservative dose, wait to give it a chance to work and then, if necessary, repeat injections until desired anesthetic level is achieved.

[a] Spinals should be placed below where the spinal cord ends (usually L1 in an adult, lower in a child); epidural location depends on the region to be anesthetized.

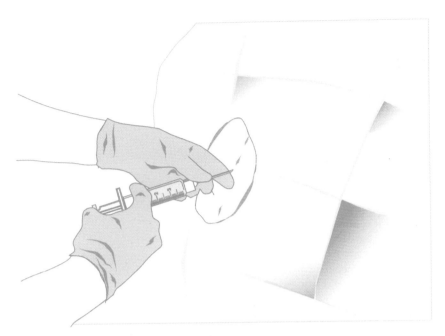

Fig. 4.6 Technique of neuraxial block placement. In this case the epidural space is sought with a "loss of resistance" technique, noting when the fluid in the syringe is suddenly easily injected.

that needle and into the intrathecal space for injection of drug. The spinal needle is withdrawn, and the epidural catheter threaded as above.

Indications

Many factors must be considered including location of operation and, therefore, anesthetic level required, duration of surgery, and implications for cardiovascular and respiratory function. For example, we would not use spinal anesthesia in a patient in hemorrhagic shock or with significant aortic stenosis who would not tolerate a drop in preload and afterload (Table 4.5).

Peripheral nerve blocks

With neuraxial anesthesia, it is difficult to block only the area of interest. Almost by definition, surgical anesthesia at the desired level includes everything "south" as well. Peripheral nerve blocks provide an alternative, interrupting nerve impulses at specific points in their course, rather than the entire spinal cord. Table 4.6 lists some of the blocks we perform.

While local anesthetics can diffuse a small distance, depositing the drug in close proximity to the desired nerve increases the likelihood of a successful block. Therefore, knowledge of anatomy is paramount. Sometimes, anatomic landmarks

Table 4.5. Indications and contraindications for neuraxial anesthesia

Indications

Surgical anesthesia, particularly below the umbilicus, and especially where consciousness is desired, e.g., obstetrics

Post-operative pain management

Labor analgesia

Chronic pain management

Contraindications

Patient refusal/inability to cooperate

Elevated intracranial pressure (risk of herniation)

Infection at site

Inadequate volume status

Coagulopathy[a]

[a] For recommendations on management of patients taking anticoagulants see www.anest.ufl.edu/EA.

Table 4.6. Indications for peripheral nerve blocks

Peripheral nerve block	Indication
Cervical plexus	Carotid endarterectomy
Stellate ganglion	Complex regional pain syndrome (CRPS) of the upper extremity (also called reflex sympathetic dystrophy, RSD)
Upper extremity	
Brachial plexus	Shoulder, arm, wrist, hand procedures
Distal nerves (median, radial, ulnar)	Forearm, hand procedures
Digital nerves	Fingers – do not use epinephrine-containing local anesthetics in finger and toe blocks. Vasoconstriction of digital arteries can lead to distal necrosis!
Intercostals	Rib fractures or chest tube placement
Celiac plexus	Chronic pain in abdomen, especially pancreatic cancer
Lumbar plexus	Lower extremity procedures
Lower extremity	
Femoral, obturator, lateral femoral cutaneous	Procedures of the thigh and knee
Sciatic and saphenous	Lower leg, calf, ankle, foot procedures
Ankle	Foot procedures

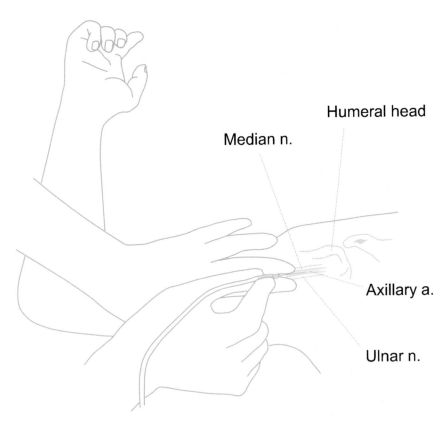

Median n.

Humeral head

Axillary a.

Ulnar n.

Fig. 4.7 Brachial plexus block: transarterial approach. We enlist an assistant to aspirate continuously on a syringe attached to the tubing. As we advance the needle, we look for aspiration of axillary arterial blood. Then we advance the needle through the back wall of the vessel and deposit local anesthetic into the axillary sheath. As we withdraw the needle, we inject an additional volume of local in the anterior sheath. Throughout the procedure, our assistant intermittently aspirates to ensure we haven't slipped the needle back into the vessel.

suffice; for example, we can deposit local anesthetic in the axillary sheath by traversing its artery (Fig. 4.7). For most other blocks, in order to ensure the needle tip lies within millimeters of the intended nerve (and not *in* the nerve), we use one of two common techniques:

(i) Paresthesia technique, in which placement of a needle in close proximity to a nerve causes a "pins and needles" sensation in the nerve's peripheral distribution. Depending on the area of the intended block, specific paresthesias can be sought with manipulation of the needle. This technique can be uncomfortable for the patient, yet requires the patient to be sufficiently awake to respond. We need to watch the patient while gauging the pressure we apply to the plunger of the syringe. The patient will let us know if he feels an "electric shock" or pain – signs we associate with the intraneural placement of the needle, at which point we do not proceed to inject drug under high pressure, which would compress the nerve in its sheath, causing nerve ischemia and injury.

(ii) Nerve stimulator technique, in which we apply a small electrical current to an insulated needle, causing motor stimulation when near a nerve. We adjust the needle position to achieve the maximal motor response in the desired distribution. This technique enables us to exploit anatomical cues to direct needle movement. For example, stimulation of the phrenic nerve (the patient will hiccup) when performing an interscalene block tells us the brachial plexus lies just a centimeter lower in the neck.

Indications

Peripheral nerve blocks may be performed for operative procedures, as well as for post-operative pain management. Through blockade of nerve impulses, pre-emptive analgesia may be obtained. Furthermore, catheter techniques enable post-operative pain management with continuous infusions of local anesthetic and/or opioids. Such infusions can improve perfusion to the operative extremity, reduce pain with movement, speed recovery, and improve quality of life even weeks after the operation.

Intravenous regional anesthesia (IVRA)

Also called a Bier[2] block, this is perhaps the simplest, safest, most foolproof regional anesthetic technique. We replace the blood in the venous system of an extremity with local anesthetic (large volume, low concentration, i.e., 0.5% lidocaine WITHOUT epinephrine) by first exsanguinating the extremity (usually arm), applying a tourniquet, then infusing the local anesthetic distal to the tourniquet. We obtain excellent anesthesia within minutes. It will last until the tourniquet is deflated. The local anesthetic will flow retrograde through the venous system into the *vasa nervorum* that bathes each nerve fiber. Unfortunately, not infrequently the patient will be troubled by tourniquet pain. Therefore, this technique is best suited for operations lasting less than an hour. The technique is safe as long as the tourniquet holds tight, preventing the local anesthetic from gaining access to the circulation and causing systemic toxicity. If the local anesthetic has been in the extremity for at least 20–30 minutes when the operation is complete, the tourniquet can be safely deflated without toxic effects.

Local anesthetic toxicity

Local anesthetics exhibit dose-related toxicity. Therefore, concerns about potential toxicity grow with increasing doses of local anesthetic (see also Pharmacology). Typical volumes of local anesthetics used for various blocks follow (we use lidocaine 1.5% as an example):

Subarachnoid block	5 mL
Epidural block (with epinephrine)	15 mL
Brachial plexus block (with epinephrine)	30 mL
Intercostal block (multiple levels)	20 mL
Finger block (*without* epinephrine)	3 mL

Of these, intercostal nerve blocks lead to the highest local anesthetic blood levels and therefore are most likely to cause toxicity, because multiple small depots of the local anesthetic offer a relatively large surface for absorption of the drug into blood vessels. In order to reduce the rate of absorption, we often add 1:200 000 epinephrine (5 mcg/mL) to the local anesthetic, which not only reduces the absorption of the drug and thus the chance of toxicity, but also prolongs the anesthetic effect.

An added advantage of the epinephrine: should the injection be inadvertently intravascular (as into an epidural vein), the prompt development of epinephrine-induced tachycardia will give a clear signal.

Either an inadvertent intravascular injection or rapid absorption of properly placed local anesthetic can trigger toxic manifestations. We reduce this risk by dividing the dose into multiple smaller boluses, looking for signs of toxicity in-between. Early typical symptoms include a metallic taste, ringing in the ears, and tingling around the mouth. Sleepiness or mental status changes often accompany these symptoms. Central nervous system toxicity progresses to seizures (treated with *small* intravenous doses of thiopental or a benzodiazepine) and eventual coma. Cardiovascular effects include hypotension due to vasodilation and myocardial depression, but may progress to complete cardiovascular collapse. This is particularly true with bupivacaine, whose slow unbinding from sodium receptors causes stubborn ventricular arrhythmias. However, eventually the drug will give way. Therefore, do not give up on resuscitative efforts.

As with all emergencies, the treatment includes the common sense steps, such as to stop injecting and then to follow the standard ABCs of basic life support. "A" (airway) and "B" (breathing with oxygen) are particularly important since hypoxia and acidosis worsen the toxicity. It sounds obvious, but do not use lidocaine to treat local anesthetic-induced ventricular arrhythmias! Use amiodarone (start with 1mg/kg slowly i.v.) instead.

Anesthesiologists skilled in both regional and general techniques offer patients a broad range of options for their operation. Regional anesthesia occupies a niche in outpatient surgery, where rapid awakening and minimal nausea/vomiting are sought. In many procedures, regional with light general anesthesia provides good operative conditions for the surgeon and excellent postoperative analgesia. Regional anesthesia plays a growing role in postoperative pain management for outpatients and for the care of some patients with chronic pain.

NOTES

1. There are many needles used for insertion of an epidural catheter, they tend to be large (to accommodate a 20 g or larger catheter), slightly blunt (to reduce the risk of dural puncture) and with a curved tip (to encourage the catheter to pass into the epidural space). Common designs include the Tuohy (introduced by Edward Boyce Tuohy (pronounced "Too-ee") around 1945) and the Weiss (designed by Jess Bernard Weiss around 1961). The latter is basically a Tuohy needle with wings at the hub.
2. August Karl Gustav Bier (1861–1949), a German surgeon, introduced intravenous regional anesthesia in 1908. He also administered and received the first spinal anesthetics in 1898 (and experienced one of the first post-dural puncture headaches the next day).

5

General anesthesia

General anesthesia requires many preparatory steps. These include the pre-operative evaluation of the patient and the procurement and preparation of all equipment to be used, drugs to be given, intravenous cannulae to be inserted for the infusion of the necessary fluids, monitors, and the tools and techniques needed for the establishment of an open airway. Elsewhere in this book you will find all of these topics addressed. Here, we will limit ourselves to a discussion of how to induce and maintain general anesthesia and how to ease the patient out of the drug-induced coma before transfer to the post-anesthesia care unit (PACU).

Induction, maintenance and emergence

Once the preparations for general anesthesia are complete, the patient's history and physical examination are reviewed, the machine and equipment are set up and tested, the patient is on the table, and the monitors are applied, we are ready to send the patient on one of the strangest journeys of his life: general anesthesia. We will administer drugs by injection and inhalation that will take possession of the patient's body. If we have used neuromuscular blocking agents, ventilation will cease, and the patient will be unable to move. In short, such an unconscious patient will have been reduced to a physiologic organism without a will.

To appreciate the enormity of this statement, consider the extreme of this condition: once general anesthesia has been established for some cardiac procedures, we might lower the patient's temperature to the point where all currently monitored variables cease to show evidence of life. There will be no heartbeat, no electrocardiogram, no spontaneous breathing, and the electroencephalogram will show no deflection. There will be no reflex, no motion, and no reaction to any intervention. If, at this point, you were to bring in an observer, unaware of what had been done, he might well pronounce the patient dead. And yet, if we raise the temperature and initiate mechanical ventilation, the patient's cardiac and respiratory function will slowly resume their own life and, once the temperature approaches normal and the effects of drugs wear off, the patient will wake up. You might ask searching questions about the patient's state, his personality, his soul during this approach to death. We cannot imagine a more profound responsibility than that of the anesthesiologist taking a patient to such an extreme approximation to death while guarding his life.

In routine general anesthesia we do not drive the system to the just described extreme. Yet, a defenseless patient under general anesthesia will expect the anesthesiologist to stand in for him and his dignity and attend to him with focused attention and great skill.

During general anesthesia, we must provide the patient with sleep, amnesia, and analgesia; we must monitor his vital signs and keep them within physiologic limits, and we must make the surgeon's task as easy as possible with the double benefit of helping the surgeon so that she can do her best for the patient. But before we start general anesthesia, an intravenous infusion (usually Ringer's lactate) is running, and we often give intravenously an anxiolytic with amnesic power such as midazolam[1] (1 to 2 mg for the average adult) and/or a narcotic, such as fentanyl (50 to 100 mcg for the average adult). Some like to give the narcotic even though the patient has no pain and even though the drug will not cause euphoria. Instead, it can serve as a gentle background and preemptive analgesic for the operation and, by weakening (but not eliminating) the sympathetic response, it can smooth out swings of blood pressure and heart rate during intubation. We always keep in mind the synergistic respiratory depression of a mixture of benzodiazepines and opioids.

Pre-oxygenation

The establishment of a patent airway is probably our most important safety concern. Disaster overtakes the patient within a matter of minutes if he cannot breathe for himself (because we paralyzed him), and we cannot ventilate his lungs (because his airway is obstructed by soft tissue and because we cannot intubate his trachea for any number of reasons). Then minutes, even seconds, count. If, before inducing apnea, we replace the nitrogen in his lungs with oxygen, we can gain 3 to 6 minutes (more with a large functional residual capacity (FRC)) before arterial hypoxemia occurs. Therefore, we routinely pre-oxygenate patients before inducing anesthesia. This procedure is simple: we apply a face mask and select a flow of oxygen high enough to prevent the patient from inhaling his exhaled nitrogen. The latter is vented and, after about 3 minutes, the patient's FRC will contain very little nitrogen, much oxygen, and the usual amount of water vapor and carbon dioxide.

Induction

We now introduce hypnotic, analgesic, and anesthetic drugs into the body either by intravenous injection or via the lungs (in the past intramuscularly or even rectally). While inhalation anesthesia can be induced without the help of intravenous drugs, the most common approach is to inject a fast-acting drug such as thiopental (3 to 5 mg/kg) or propofol (1 to 3 mg/kg). Within a couple of minutes, these drugs will reach their peak effect, at which time intubation of the trachea becomes feasible, usually with the help of muscle relaxants such as succinylcholine. Neither thiopental nor propofol offers relaxation of muscles or analgesia. Therefore, they are wonderful for gentle induction but would be unlikely to provide adequate operating conditions for an intra-abdominal procedure.

Instead of intubating the trachea, we have the option of inserting a laryngeal mask airway (LMA), which does not require the use of a muscle relaxant and is particularly welcome when the patient need not be intubated at all and is breathing spontaneously throughout the operation (see Airway management chapter).

Once we have placed the endotracheal tube or LMA and have confirmed its proper location by auscultation and end-tidal CO_2, we can begin the administration of inhalation, intravenous (TIVA, total intravenous anesthesia) or a combination anesthetic. A number of halogenated drugs are available (halothane, isoflurane, desflurane, sevoflurane), but we use only one at a time. Each can be given together with 50–70% nitrous oxide in oxygen. Nitrous oxide provides modest analgesic background without cardiovascular depression to speak of. Surgical anesthesia (the patient will not respond to the incision) can be obtained within a matter of minutes so that the induction of anesthesia need not delay the incision.

Propofol is the poster child agent for TIVA. Purported advantages of this technique are shortened wake-up and PACU times, and reduced risk of postoperative nausea and vomiting. Rather than halogenated agents, patients for outpatient surgery might receive a propofol infusion (for sedation and sleep) with nitrous oxide to provide a modicum of analgesia and ensure amnesia, supplemented with small amounts of analgesics.

The rapid sequence induction

Patients who need general anesthesia, even though they have a full stomach (having recently eaten or having a condition that interferes with gastric emptying such as trauma or pregnancy), require a special technique, the so-called rapid sequence induction (Table 5.1). With a full stomach, the specter of regurgitation and aspiration arises. The technique calls for a thorough denitrogenation, followed by the administration of thiopental and succinylcholine in rapid succession while we maintain pressure on the cricoid ring (the so-called Sellick maneuver[2]). Remember, the cricoid is the only ring of the trachea that does not have a membrane posteriorly and, instead, is cartilaginous throughout its circumference. So, pushing on it compresses the esophagus. You can feel the cricoid ring just under the larynx. Only once we have confirmed the proper position of the endotracheal tube and inflated the cuff can we stop the Sellick maneuver.

Table 5.1. Steps in a rapid sequence induction

Once you have started a rapid sequence induction, you have lost the opportunity to check or obtain missing equipment. Thorough preparation therefore, is mandatory.

Preparation

1. Prepare and check for function:
   * suction
   * intubation equipment
     * tubes – one too large, one just right, one too small – check cuffs
     * laryngoscope – two different blades – check lights
   * machine
   * emergency cricothyrotomy set available
2. Have available a helper skilled in applying cricoid pressure and to assist as necessary
3. Prepare patient
   * give antacid if circumstance permits
   * obtain vital signs, print ECG strip

Induction

1. Pre-oxygenate/de-nitrogenate to an end-tidal oxygen of 80 to 90%
2. Tell the patient he will feel pressure on his neck as he falls asleep; meanwhile the assistant gently locates the cricoid ring
3. In rapid succession, administer an intubating dose of thiopental (or propofol) followed by an intubating dose of succinylcholine, while the assistant begins to apply cricoid pressure (20 newtons)
4. As patient falls asleep, assistant increases cricoid pressure (40 newtons)
5. Sixty seconds after the succinylcholine entered the vein (or when apnea and relaxation coincide), intubate the trachea under direct laryngoscopy
6. Connect endotracheal tube to breathing circuit, inflate the cuff of the endotracheal tube then inflate the lung
7. Confirm endotracheal position of tube by
   * watching chest rise – bilaterally
   * listening for breath sounds – bilaterally in axillae
   * listening over stomach for absence of breath sounds
   * observing capnogram for appearance of carbon dioxide for 6 breaths.
8. Tell assistant to release cricoid pressure after confirming correct position of the tube
9. Secure tube and begin anesthesia

Positioning

For many operations, the patient can lie on his back. Others require positions that may take an hour or more to be accomplished (for example, neurosurgical operations). We need to understand what position favors access for the surgeon and what positions present dangers for the patient (interference with ventilation, compression of nerves, extreme flexion or extension of joints). Thus, the positioning is often a joint surgical/anesthesia task during which a lot of foam padding finds application between patient and hard surfaces. The most common post-operative nerve palsy affects the ulnar nerve (funny bone), which is exposed to pressure, being superficial and running through the ulnar groove at the elbow (between the medial epicondyle and the olecranon).

Depth of anesthesia and monitoring

Once the patient is positioned, we must keep the anesthetic level so that the patient will neither feel pain nor remember the operation. Yet this "anesthetic depth" must be balanced against the hemodynamic consequences (hypotension) of excess anesthetic, as well as the potential for delayed wake-up. If the patient is not paralyzed, there will be little doubt that he will move and let us know if he feels pain. We need to gauge the depth of anesthesia clinically and with the help of instruments. The clinical assessment includes monitoring heart rate and blood pressure, which should be neither high from sympathetic response to noxious stimulation, nor low from overdose with anesthetics. In recent years processed EEG signals have become available that claim to help gauge the depth of anesthesia by generating a score linked to EEG activity, which becomes depressed as anesthesia deepens. In addition to these signals we keep track of the intravenous drugs the patient has had, of their effects and duration, and of the concentration of expired anesthetics, which reflect blood and finally brain levels. Thus the conduct of general anesthesia calls for continual attention to a number of parameters and variables.

At the same time, we monitor pulse oximetry, blood pressure, heart rate, ECG, tidal volume, respiratory rate and peak inspiratory pressure, inspired oxygen, the concentration of respired gases and vapors, and the capnogram. Should blood loss, deep anesthesia, surgical activity (for example compressing the vena cava), an embolism (for example, air aspirated in an open vein), or a process originating in the patient (such as anaphylaxis or coronary insufficiency) cause a problem, we should be able to discover the effects as early as possible so that we can take corrective actions. We also assess the degree of muscle relaxation with the help of a nerve stimulator (twitch monitor) and by watching the operation and gauging muscle tone, which might impede the surgeon's work. Thus, we cannot be satisfied with watching the monitors; we need to keep an eye on the patient, his face, his position, and the surgeon's work.

A tedious aspect of our work is the obligation to keep a record of all these events and of our activities, such as the administration of drugs and fluids, adjustment of ventilator settings, and even of surgical events ("aorta clamped at 9:24 am!"). Automated record keeping systems are becoming increasingly sophisticated.

Emergence

Well before the surgeon puts in the last stitch, we begin preparation for having the patient wake up. This might call for the reversal of a non-depolarizing neuromuscular blocking drug and the scaling back of inspired anesthetic concentrations. Furthermore, our goal is to have the patient awaken quickly and without pain; therefore, we titrate opioids or our regional anesthetic to anticipate the pain level without unacceptable respiratory depression, while also considering the risk for postoperative nausea and vomiting. It is a fine art to gauge the surgical process and the patient's requirements so that the patient opens his eyes when the dressing goes on. "Hello," we say, and, after confirming the patient is strong, able to protect his airway (gag reflex), breathing and following commands, we suction his airway and say, "All done! Let me take out that tube," when we pull the endotracheal tube or the LMA. While the patient is not likely to remember such words, they provide a fitting ending to a perfect anesthetic!

We then accompany the patient to the Post-Anesthesia Care Unit (PACU) where we go through a formal process of turning the care of the patient over to a specialized PACU nurse, unless the patient is fit for early discharge home or needs to be admitted to the Intensive Care Unit.

Problems

Things don't always run smoothly. If critical incidents occur, they must be discovered and corrected in time, lest they lead to disasters. To catch early trends, however, presents more difficulties than one might think, because most signals we monitor are rather non-specific. Thus, a low SpO_2 could be the result of malignant hyperthermia or faulty hospital piping, or low blood pressure the consequence of bleeding, deep anesthesia, or a measuring artifact. Therefore, with any deviation from normal, we need to think holistically about the patient and the anesthesia system with all of its components.

In Table 5.2, we have listed trends in various monitored parameters as they often appear during certain problems. Observe two points:

(i) Usually we cannot arrive at a diagnosis by simply looking at the monitors. We need additional information, which we must urgently collect when trends herald trouble.

(ii) Breath and heart sounds turn out to be very helpful. Always listen to heart and lungs (wheezing, crackling, uneven breath sounds – or, importantly – normal breath sounds) to include or exclude certain items from a differential diagnosis. Equally important is the peak inspiratory pressure.

To complicate matters even further, not all patients react in an identical manner. Co-existing diseases can obscure changes or reverse direction of an expected change. Finally, trends can reverse direction, depending on how long the problem existed and how grave the incident. For example, hypercarbia and hypoxemia secondary to inadequate ventilation because of obstruction in the endotracheal tube can first cause sympathetic stimulation and a rise in blood pressure and heart rate. However, if the problem persists, pressure will decline and, with severe hypoxemia, extreme bradycardia can supervene.

Table 5.2. Likely initial direction of trends of commonly monitored signals in patients under general anesthesia with mechanical ventilation[a]

Problem	BP	HR	SpO$_2$	ETCO$_2$	PIP	Breath sounds
Breathing system obstruction	Up	Up	Down	Down	Up	Abnormal
Transfusion reaction	Down	Up	Down	Down	Up	Abnormal
Anaphylaxis	Down	Up	Down	Down	Up	Abnormal
Pulmonary edema	Down	Up	Down	Down	Up	Abnormal
Aspiration		Up	Down	Down	Up	Abnormal
Asthma		Up	Down	Down	Up	Abnormal
Myocardial infarction	Down	Up	Down	Down		Abnormal with edema
Cardiac tamponade	Down	Up	Down	Down		Normal
Pulmonary embolism	Down	Up	Down	Down		Normal
Hemorrhage	Down	Up		Down		Normal
Esophageal intubation	Up	Up	Down	Absent		Abnormal
Light anesthesia	Up	Up				Normal
Malignant hyperthermia	Up	Up	Down	Up		Normal
Disconnect	Up	Up	Down	Absent	Down	Abnormal
Endobronchial intubation		Up	Down	Down	Up	Abnormal
Pneumothorax	Down	Up	Down	Down	Up	Abnormal
Addison crisis	Down	Up		Down		Normal

[a] These may vary with severity, duration and the patient's condition.

BP: blood pressure, HR: heart rate, SpO$_2$: oxyhemoglobin saturation, ETCO$_2$: end-tidal carbon dioxide, PIP: peak inspiratory pressure.

Malignant hyperthermia: Patients with this rare ($\approx$1:20 000) inherited defect in intracellular calcium control are asymptomatic until given succinylcholine or anesthetic vapors, which can trigger a violent increase in metabolism with skyrocketing O$_2$ consumption and CO$_2$ production. Tachycardia and rapidly rising ETCO$_2$ precede by many minutes a murderous fever. High creatine kinase levels reflect extensive muscle damage. Immediate cooling and i.v. dantrolene have greatly improved the prognosis. Triggering agents must be avoided subsequently.

NOTES

1. Please consult the Pharmacology chapter for details on the drugs mentioned.
2. Brian A. Sellick (1918–1996) – a British anesthetist who made numerous contributions in cardiothoracic anesthesia, is best known for a seminal paper describing cricoid pressure to prevent gastric reflux and distension from mask–ventilation.

6

Post-operative care

The post-operative care of the patient can be divided into an early and a continued phase. The early phase lasts from the moment the patient leaves the operating room until he is discharged from the Post-Anesthesia Care Unit (PACU) or its equivalent. The care is then continued, a phase that can extend for days or even weeks.

Early post-operative care

Based on his medical condition and the planned operative procedure, we will have classified the patient as ambulatory (also known as outpatient), as 'post-operative admit' (the patient comes to the hospital on the day of the operation and is admitted to the hospital after his operation), or as an inpatient (the patient is already in the hospital, or will be admitted for pre-operative preparation, and will stay there post-operatively). Two categories of patients might bypass the PACU (formerly called the Recovery Room): (i) ambulatory patients who had a minor procedure and are expected to be ready for discharge in a matter of minutes and (ii) patients requiring intensive care because of serious pre-operative medical problems or major operations with potential complications. Such patients are admitted directly to the Intensive Care Unit (ICU) upon completion of the operation.

For patients coming to the PACU we consider three factors: the patient's pre-operative condition; the effects of the just completed therapeutic (surgical, radiological, obstetrical, electroconvulsive) or diagnostic procedure; and the effects of the anesthetic. As we turn the patient's care over to the PACU staff, we provide a formal "report" of his condition including the following:

- pre-existing medical conditions with particular emphasis on pre-existing respiratory, cardiac, and chronic pain issues;
- surgical disease, operative and anesthetic course, and any problems encountered;
- fluid status including what was administered, estimated blood loss, and urine output;

- medications administered in the operating room. We mention antagonists given to counteract lingering neuromuscular weakness or respiratory depression or nausea and vomiting. Should the patient need more such medication, the PACU physician can either continue the already initiated treatment or, if the patient does not respond, switch to another drug;
- concerns regarding the procedure or the patient, including the plan for post-operative pain management;
- issues requiring follow-up such as pending laboratory evaluations or a chest radiograph to confirm central venous catheter placement.

Finally, we make certain the patient is stable, record a first set of vital signs obtained in the PACU, and ensure that all documentation is complete and correct.

In the PACU, we first worry about safety. We consider waning anesthetic drug effects as they relate to adequacy of oxygenation, which in turn requires an alert respiratory center (is there a hangover effect from CNS depressants?) and the muscle power to breathe (is there a hangover effect from muscle relaxants or a regional anesthetic?), an open airway (is there obstruction of the upper airway?), and no encumbrance to breathing from dressing, position, or the surgical procedure. Adequacy of oxygenation also requires adequate circulation (is the blood pressure normal and the ECG unchanged from its preoperative state?). The pulse oximeter will speak volumes to these questions. If the patient is *breathing room air* and his oxygenation (as measured by pulse oximetry located peripherally) is normal, we can be assured of adequate breathing.

We assess the central nervous system, recognizing that the patient usually will have had a number of drugs with CNS effects. With modern anesthetic techniques and drugs, we expect the patient to rally from the depressant effects of the drugs fairly rapidly and to become responsive, if not immediately oriented. Up to 25% of elderly patients will be delirious after a general anesthetic for a major surgical procedure. Once a patient is not only responsive but also oriented, we know that his brain is perfused and oxygenated.

Most patients will arrive with an intravenous infusion. If we assume that the patient is in a neutral fluid balance (blood pressure and urine output back to preoperative values), in short, if his insensible losses (about 800 mL/day) and intra-operative losses (from evaporation from exposed surfaces, e.g., intestines, bleeding and from edema caused by the surgical trauma (the so-called third space or blister)) have been replaced, fluid therapy will simply continue to replace insensible losses following the 4–2–1 rule (see Table 6.1).

Often enough, however, some bleeding continues – usually invisibly – into the traumatized tissue. Fluid therapy will need to be adjusted to meet the patient's requirements as judged by cardiovascular signs and urine production. A balanced salt solution such as normal saline or Ringer's lactate will serve as long as there is no need to worry about electrolytes, red blood cells, and plasma proteins.

Table 6.1. The 4–2–1 rule for fluid maintenance based on body weight[a]

Body weight	Fluid administration
For the first 10 kg	4 mL/kg/h
For the next 10 kg	Add 2 mL/kg/h
For each kg above 20 kg	Add 1 mL/kg/h

[a] For a 70 kg man this would amount to $40 + 20 + 50 =$ 110 mL/h for the duration of fasting.

Early post-operative pain

As we reassure ourselves as to the patient's safety, we begin to consider the patient's pain. Three points need attention: (i) surgical incisional pain will decrease over time, (ii) analgesic effects left over from the anesthetic will wane over time, and (iii) pain counteracts the CNS depressant (respiratory) effects of narcotic analgesics (Fig. 6.1). Thus, pain management in the PACU must seek a balance of three shifting slopes of which we do not know the rate of change. This translates into: *watch the patient* and titrate drugs to balance adequate analgesia and avoid respiratory depression. As long as the patient cannot take oral medication, a practical approach for the acute phase of pain management in the PACU can make use of intravenous morphine in 2.0 mg increments for the average adult. It takes about 5 minutes for such a dose to show an effect. Therefore, wait at least 5 minutes before giving the next dose. Many factors influence the patient's response to such treatment. A patient on chronic narcotic therapy will require more, a frail elderly person less. Titrate! Titrate! Titrate!

After minor surgical procedures, many patients will not require opioids at all, and most can take oral medication. The pharmacology chapter gives drugs and dosages.

There would be no need for a PACU if it were not for the occasional complications that require early recognition and prompt treatment. Here is a quick review of potential problems encountered in the PACU.

Complications

Desaturation
Differential diagnosis

- *Hypoventilation Always first assist ventilation to establish normal SpO_2 and $PaCO_2$!* Then consider causes and their treatment.

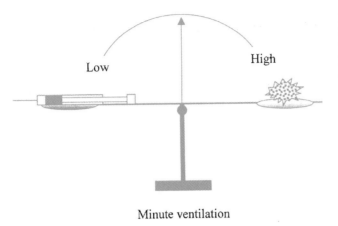

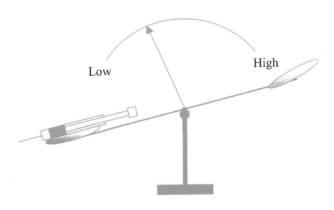

Fig. 6.1 Ventilatory response to PaCO$_2$. The first diagram shows that noxious stimulation (spiked beasty on the right) can counteract the respiratory depressant effect of narcotics (syringe), maintaining a normal ventilatory response to PaCO$_2$. In the lower diagram the pain has vanished and the respiratory depressant effect of the narcotic becomes unmasked, minute ventilation is low. Such depression can even result in apnea.

- *Residual neuromuscular blockade* Suspected when the patient shows an abnormal respiratory pattern, particularly the tracheal tug, i.e., downward motion of the larynx with inspiration. Test with the twitch monitor. Treat with reversal agents.
- *Residual sedation* Consider reversal of benzodiazepines with flumazenil.
- *Narcosis* Typically a slow, deep respiratory pattern; consider cautious reversal of opioids with naloxone.
- *Bronchospasm (wheezing)* Intubation is a strong stimulant for bronchospasm; treat with bronchodilators.
- *Laryngospasm (stridor)* If related to the operation, e.g., neck operation with possible hematoma formation, it becomes a surgical emergency. Try continuous positive airway pressure, letting the patient exhale against resistance (5 to 10 cmH$_2$O) and maintaining that pressure throughout the respiratory cycle.

- *Pain* Particularly with a subcostal incision where deep breathing is painful.
- *Ventilation/Perfusion mismatch*
  - *Atelectasis* Probably the most common cause of post-operative hypoxemia.
  - *Aspiration of gastric contents* Particularly in high-risk patients, or if intubation required multiple attempts.
  - *Pneumothorax* Especially after central venous access. Obtain a chest radiograph, but be prepared to relieve the pneumothorax by puncture (2nd intercostal space, mid-clavicular line) should a tension pneumothorax develop in the meantime.
  - *Pulmonary embolism* Thromboembolism is the most common. May need V/Q or CT scanning. Most surgical patients require some form of prophylaxis against deep vein thrombosis (DVT).
  - *Pneumonia*
  - *Mainstem intubation*
- *Diffusion block*
  - *Pulmonary edema*
- *Inadequate FiO$_2$*

Management

(i) Airway
  - Chin lift, neck extension; continuous positive airway pressure (CPAP) often helps. For this, use a bag and mask system (Mapleson – see The anesthesia machine) with a high flow (15 L/min) of oxygen. Apply the face mask tightly, letting the patient exhale against resistance (5 to 10 cmH$_2$O) and maintain that pressure throughout the respiratory cycle.

(ii) Breathing
  - Supplemental oxygen
    - Via nasal cannula, but with oxygen flows of 2 L/min the inspired O$_2$ only increases by about 6%.
    - Via standard tent face mask for an inspired O$_2$ of up to 50%
    - Via partial rebreathing face mask for an inspired O$_2$ of up to 80%
    - Via non-rebreathing face mask for an inspired O$_2$ of up to 95%
  - Encouragement – "take a breath!" often effective with narcotic depression
  - Bag–Mask – use with self-inflating bag or Mapleson
  - Check ventilator settings, O$_2$ supply and end-tidal CO$_2$ if the patient is intubated.

(iii) Studies to consider
  - Chest radiograph if abnormal breath sounds (pneumonia, atelectasis, pneumothorax, +/− aspiration). Keep in mind, however, that a portable film may not provide the highest quality and consolidation takes some time to manifest radiographically.

- Arterial blood gas
- Twitch monitor if patient appears to be partially paralyzed.

Hypotension
Differential diagnosis
- Inadequate preload
  - Inadequate fluid resuscitation
  - Continued hemorrhage
  - Venodilation due to medications or sympathetic blockade
  - Pericardial tamponade
  - Pulmonary embolism
  - Increased intra-abdominal pressure, e.g., big uterus pressing on vena cava
  - Increased intra-thoracic pressure, e.g., tension pneumothorax
- Poor contractility
  - Residual anesthetics
  - Myocardial ischemia
  - Fluid overload ("far-side" of the Starling Curve)
  - Pre-existing cardiac dysfunction
  - Electrolyte disturbance
  - Hypothermia
- Inadequate afterload
  - Sepsis
  - Vasodilation due to medications or sympathetic blockade, e.g., neuraxial anesthetic
  - Anaphylaxis
- Arrhythmias
  - Bradycardia
  - Loss of atrial kick
    - Atrial fibrillation/flutter
    - AV dissociation
  - Electrolyte disturbance

Management
- Physical examination (especially chest auscultation)
- ECG (at least 5-lead strip) to detect arrhythmias and ischemia
- ACLS protocol if abnormal rhythm
- Hemoglobin level
- Intravascular fluid resuscitation +/− blood transfusion
- Supplemental oxygen
- Elevate legs to enhance venous return
- Consider transthoracic echo
- Consider chest radiograph

- Consider invasive monitoring
- Check electrolytes, especially Ca^{2+} for inotropy and K^+, Mg^{2+} for arrhythmias

Hypertension

Differential diagnosis

- Pain
- Pre-existing hypertension
- Bladder distension
- Rebound hypertension (especially with chronic clonidine)
- Endocrine problem (thyroid storm, pheochromocytoma)
- Malignant hyperthermia
- Delirium tremens
- Increased intracranial pressure

Management

- Treat pain or anxiety if present.
- Review for pre-existing hypertension and reinstitute anti-hypertensive therapy where appropriate.
- Check ECG.
- Look for additional signs of malignant hyperthermia.
- Check for high bladder dome. If Foley catheter in place, check patency, or perform in-and-out catheterization.

We hope that none of these problems arose or that they have been dealt with successfully, at which point we are ready to discharge the patient from the PACU.

PACU discharge

A frequently used checklist is the Aldrete Recovery Score (see Table 6.2). If the sum of points reaches 9 or 10, we can discharge the patient from the PACU.

Outpatients

After outpatient procedures under local or peripheral nerve block anesthesia, perhaps with parenterally administered CNS depressants, e.g., midazolam (Versed®), propofol or opioids, the patient may bypass the PACU unless a medical condition would call for observation. It may be necessary to prescribe an oral analgesic that might include a mild opioid.

If no CNS depressant drug was used during the procedure and if the peripheral nerve block is behaving as expected (surgical anesthesia wearing off, but perhaps analgesia continuing), the patient can be discharged. We still insist that a relative or friend accompany them home because the patient will have been exposed to the stress of an operation – however minor – and will have been fasting and thus be at risk of swooning or even fainting and not being at the height of his reflex responses.

Table 6.2. Aldrete score for post-anesthesia recovery[a]

System	Description	Score
Activity	Able to move four extremities voluntarily or on command	2
	Able to move two extremities voluntarily or on command	1
	Unable to move voluntarily or on command	0
Respiration	Able to breathe deeply and cough freely	2
	Dyspnea or limited breathing	1
	Apneic	0
Circulation	Blood pressure +/− 20% of pre-anesthetic values	2
	Blood pressure +/− 20–49% of pre-anesthetic values	1
	Blood pressure +/− 50% of pre-anesthetic values	0
Consciousness	Fully awake	2
	Arousable on calling	1
	Non-responsive	0
Oxygenation	Able to maintain saturation >90% on room air	2
	Needs oxygen to maintain saturation >90%	1
	Saturation <90% even with oxygen	0

Aldrete J.A. The post-anesthesia recovery score revisited (letter). *J. Clin. Anesth.* 1995;7:89.

[a] A score of 9 or 10 suggests the patient is stable for discharge from the PACU.

For those patients who required CNS depressants for a short operative procedure in which no severe post-operative pain is expected, e.g., a sigmoidoscopy under propofol sedation or a cataract removal under local anesthesia preceded by a small (0.5 to 0.75 mg/kg) dose of methohexital (Brevital®) to minimize the discomfort of the retrobulbar block, the recovery process can be completed in a matter of minutes to an hour, at which point the patient can be discharged into the care of a relative or friend for transportation home. We always assume that drug effects and hormonal disturbances will linger for a matter of several hours to a day, so that upon discharge, the patient cannot be considered ready to drive an automobile or ride a bicycle or even cross the street by himself.

For those patients who remain in the hospital following their operation, PACU discharge signals the phase of continued post-operative care.

Continued post-operative care

The patient will go through important changes in response to a major operation with anesthesia. The stress of the inflicted surgical trauma will trigger a release of adrenocorticotropic hormones, cortisol, and catecholamines. Catabolism will overpower anabolism; the patient will be in a negative nitrogen balance.

Coagulation changes might further thrombosis. Incisional pain and narcotic analgesics can reduce pulmonary gas exchange. Narcotics inhibit the cough reflex, already reduced in the elderly, causing patients to retain bronchial secretions, potentially leading to atelectasis and pneumonitis. Large fluid loads given during the operation need to be mobilized, yet antidiuretic hormone secretion will favor water and salt retention. An ileus after intra-abdominal procedures often takes days to resolve while nasogastric suction deflates the stomach not without removing electrolytes. In short, many major operations will leave the patient in a greatly debilitated state that can take several days to resolve.

If these processes are superimposed on extensive surgical operations, for example those affecting heart, lung or brain, the patient will be admitted to the ICU. This will also be true for post-operative patients who come with pre-existing disease processes involving the cardiovascular (congestive heart failure, recent myocardial infarction), or respiratory (obstructive lung disease) systems, the central nervous system (stroke, tumor), metabolism (diabetes), hepatic or renal systems, or infection. The available frequency of observation, extent of monitoring, and immediacy of care in the ICU does not match what is available in the operating room, but greatly exceeds whatever can be offered on the post-surgical ward.

When we visit the patient on the post-surgical ward, we will not only consult his chart to see the trends in vital signs (cardiovascular, respiratory and temperature) but also assess fluid status and medications prescribed and given. We then talk to the patient to gauge his mental status (up to 25% of elderly patients can take up to a week to become fully oriented, and some 10% have cognitive impairment lasting for months) and to ask about his comfort. We might have to explain that hoarseness (from an endotracheal tube) or a sore throat (from an LMA or endotracheal tube) are likely to improve in a day or two. We continue to worry about pulmonary complications, e.g., atelectasis and pneumonitis, which are most likely in elderly men, in smokers, and after operations that involve the upper abdomen and the chest. Being aware that myocardial infarctions are far more likely to occur – many of them silently – on the second post-operative day than in the operating room, we pay special attention to the cardiovascular system. Hypotension, hypertension (often pre-existing), and arrhythmias are not uncommon.

Pain management

As anesthesiologists, we are particularly attentive to the patient's pain and its management. We now use a widely employed standardized method of assessing pain in adults and children (Fig. 6.2). In children incapable of relating their pain, physical signs can help (Table 6.3). The treatment of pain will be influenced by its severity.

If the patient is unable to take oral medication, we can institute patient-controlled intravenous opioid administration (PCA), a system that enables the

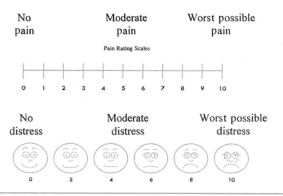

Pain assessment guide
Tell me about your pain

VAS = Pain intensity (0 - 10), patient report

If 0 is no pain and 10 is the worst pain imaginable, what is your pain now? …in the last 24 hours?

Fig. 6.2 VAS pain assessment guide. Adult patients will be asked to select a number on the visual analogue scale (VAS), while children can point to one of the faces to describe their pain.

patient to trigger an intravenous injection of a predetermined amount of a narcotic. The PCA pumps can be programmed to deliver a specific volume, then to lock the system for a predetermined period. When the patient pushes a button, a typical program might deliver (into a running intravenous drip) a 1 mL bolus containing 1.0 mg morphine. The pump then goes into a lockout mode, making an additional injection impossible for a preprogrammed period of, for example, 5 minutes. The pump can be programmed to limit the hourly injection to, for example, no more than 12 mg/h. Even that amount will be excessive if the patient were to self-administer the maximum, hour after hour. The dose and the lock-out period have to be tailored for the individual patient. While morphine is the standard, several drugs are available, among them hydromorphone (Dilaudid®) and fentanyl. In addition, for patients who pre-operatively have become tolerant to opioids, a background infusion of the narcotic may be required.

Depending on the operation (some cause much more severe and protracted pain than others; some limit oral intake for a longer period) and the patient (some are much more sensitive than others), a PCA pump might be available to the patient for a day or a week or more. Once narcotics are no longer needed, or the patient can tolerate p.o. intake, oral medications take over. A great variety of drugs are available (see Pharmacology).

Table 6.3. Pain assessment guide in children

	Pain assessment guide in children Behavioral/distress score (0–10, Caregiver) FLACC scale (face, legs, activity, cry, consolability)		
	0	1	2
Face	No particular expression or smile	Occasional grimace or frown, withdrawn, uninterested	Frequent to constant frown, clenched jaw, quivering chin
Legs	Normal position or relaxed	Uneasy, restless, tense	Kicking or legs drawn up
Activity	Lying quietly, normal position, moves easily	Squirming, shifting back/forth, tense	Arched, rigid or jerking
Cry	No cry asleep or awake	Moans or whimpers, occasional complaint	Crying steadily, screams or sobs, frequent complaints
Consolability	Content, relaxed	Reassured by occasional touching, hugging, or "talking to", distractible	Difficult to console or comfort

Some patients will still have an epidural catheter in place that had served the anesthetic management during a thoracic, abdominal or lower extremity operation and can now be used for pain management. Typically, we infuse a low concentration of local anesthetic combined with a narcotic through the catheter. By combining these drugs, we minimize the amount of motor block (paralysis) from the local anesthetic while limiting narcotic side effects (nausea, itching, and urinary retention) associated with larger doses of opioids. Once we establish a level of analgesia with a bolus injection, an infusion is begun and the patient might regulate the administration of additional drug with a PCA pump (PCEA: patient controlled epidural analgesia). Dose and concentration of local anesthetic and lock-out period will have to be adjusted for the individual patient and drugs infused. A typical arrangement might deliver 0.2 mg of morphine in 1.0 mL fluid containing 0.25% bupivacaine and a lock-out period of 10 minutes. Other approaches use a continuous epidural infusion alone.

The post-operative recovery will progress slowly. Every day, if all is going well, we can see improvements. Indeed, we can often see the moment when the patient 'turns the corner' from negative to positive nitrogen balance. He will start shaving, she will do her hair and even put on lipstick. The patient will begin to eat, and we can switch from parenteral to oral medication. Many patients will be discharged from the hospital with prescriptions for oral analgesics. See the

Pharmacology chapter for a list of commonly used drugs, dosages and duration of effect.

Chronic pain

Anesthesiologists have assumed an ever-increasing role in the treatment of patients with pain that ranges from the acute pain in the PACU, to the persisting (days rather than hours) post-operative pain, to the truly chronic (weeks and months rather than days) pain. The latter often does not arise from a surgical trauma but instead from tumors and degenerative diseases. The armamentarium of the chronic pain physician also differs from that of the acute care anesthesiologist. Gone are invasive monitors and moment-to-moment control of vital signs. Still very much in evidence are regional anesthesia procedures and a vast array of medications, most of them to be taken by mouth. Many patients with chronic pain suffer greatly from conditions for which we cannot find an anatomic explanation, conditions the treatment of which require as much skill and compassion as should be expected by a patient with traumatic pain. Thus, for all patients with chronic pain, we emphasize a dual approach: pharmacologic treatment and non-pharmacologic treatment that includes therapeutic exercises and distraction techniques and massage, which calls for the skills of nurses, physical therapists, and psychologists.

In the management of chronic pain, a number of different nerve blocks have been used. More common among them are stellate ganglion and paravertebral sympathetic blocks, e.g., for complex regional pain syndrome (CRPS), formerly called reflex sympathetic dystrophy (RSD), and celiac plexus block, e.g., for pain from pancreatic cancer. Nerve blocks are often repeated to tide the patient over a condition that can be expected to improve. If that is not the case, neurolytic (destructive) nerve blocks can be considered. For these, alcohol or phenol have been used. Such blocks are usually employed only for terminally ill cancer patients, not only because of the potential for serious side effects but also because axons often regrow with recurrence of pain in two or three months, and some patients develop a central denervation dysesthesia, which is very difficult to treat.

The first step will always be to assess the severity of pain, if for no other reason than to gauge the effectiveness of the treatment. A guideline for treatment might suggest the following:

- *For mild pain* (*VAS 4 or below*) Oral medication with acetaminophen such as tramadol/acetaminophen (Ultracet ®) is often sufficient. If necessary, we might consider low dose narcotics, such as oxycodone or hydrocodone.
- *For moderate to severe pain* (*VAS up to 7*) We would rely more on narcotics such as morphine or hydromorphone (Dilaudid®). Depending on the

circumstances, centrally acting muscle relaxants, anti-depressants, and anxi-olytics can be added.

- *For the most severe pain* Higher doses of narcotics, continuous infusions through implanted catheters, e.g., intrathecal or epidural pumps, and in terminally ill patients, neurolytic nerve blocks will come into consideration.

In the past, many patients suffered greatly because physicians feared that opiate medication would lead to addiction. Such concerns must be tempered by the obligation to alleviate pain and will be abandoned when dealing with a terminally ill patient.

7

Monitoring

Introduction

Imagine stepping into an operating room. You see a patient draped for the operation, the surgical team, the anesthesiologist, an anesthesia machine, a ventilator, one or more infusion pumps, bags with intravenous fluids, and a monitor with a screen full of curves and numbers. But the picture is not static. The people move, the bellows of the ventilator go up and down, the drip chambers of the infusion sets show drops of fluids, and on the monitor the ECG, blood pressure, SpO_2, and capnographic patterns run across the screen. You behold this scene that presents an enormous amount of continuously changing data. You also hear the surgeon asking for an instrument, the scrub nurse saying something to the circulator, the anesthesiologist conveying to the surgeon information from the patient's medical record, the ventilator puffing, and a monitor beeping. Depending on your experience, you will know how to interpret what your senses absorb. You can imagine the scene with calm professionals at work at a routine task or one with frantic activity during an emergency punctuated by the urgently sounding alarms.

In this scene, *you* are the monitor. You absorb an abundance of signals that present data, which in your mind turn into information. You turn this information into knowledge, depending on what you know about the patient, the operation, and the clinical team. This knowledge depends on information about the patient's history and, ideally, acquaintance with the patient himself. If you were to record all the facts that you can comprehend, you would wind up with a very, very long list. On paper, it would take hours to synthesize, from such a comprehensive list of facts and ever changing trends, the current status of the patient. Such knowledge would enable you to make certain statements about this moment in time and projections into the immediate future.

When you think about monitoring, please remember that the physical diagnosis – still part of monitoring in anesthesia – and the elaborate electronic monitors present only a minute fraction of the data that *you*, the clinical monitor, require and absorb in order to understand what is going on with your patient. The electronic monitors supplement in a modest way what the clinician perceives.

Let us now look at the small fraction of information generated by physical examination and by electronic and mechanical monitors.

Assume that the patient undergoes an operation under epidural anesthesia and light sedation. In addition to all the data described above, you will observe that the patient is breathing spontaneously. That means he has a heart beat and a blood pressure sufficient to perfuse his respiratory center. If the patient responds appropriately to a question, we know his brain is adequately oxygenated. Now, that is a lot of information picked up without instruments!

Now assume the patient to be under general anesthesia and paralyzed, and that a ventilator mechanically breathes for him. Without getting a little closer, you cannot know if the patient has a heart beat, a blood pressure, a perfused brain, or enough oxygen to keep the brain out of trouble. Enter focused monitoring . . .

Focused monitoring

Our goals in monitoring the patient under anesthesia are driven by two considerations:

(i) Are we ventilating the patient's lungs optimally and giving just the right amount of drugs and fluids? In other words, we monitor so that we can titrate our ministrations to a conceptual optimum.

(ii) Do the data we gather from the patient and the equipment indicate potential danger or trends that require our intervention? In other words, for safety's sake, we monitor variables that can indicate threatening problems, be they the consequence of anesthetic or surgical actions or based on the patient's disease.

Many signals we monitor subserve both titration and safety. For example, during anesthesia, we observe the patient's response to electrical stimulation of a motor nerve (the "twitch monitor") in order to *titrate* the administration of neuromuscular blocking drugs (muscle relaxants). At the end of anesthesia, we observe the same response in order to make sure that the patient has adequate muscle power to breathe without help – an important *safety concern*! Many, perhaps even most, other signals fall only into the safety category. For example, we monitor the ECG, oxygen saturation and inspired CO_2 for safety sake, not for titration.

All monitoring builds on old-fashioned inspection, auscultation, and palpation. Indeed, instruments do not tell all, and at times may even fail. The clinician must still be able to assess the patient and the system without recourse to instruments. Rarely will the instruments alone make a diagnosis for you. More often than not, you will have to take into consideration facts not captured by instruments. First comes inspection.

Inspection

More than any other monitoring activity in the operating room, inspection must be practised and honed. In anesthesia, the pattern of breathing gives more important information than any other observation.

Spontaneous ventilation

During spontaneous breathing, the patient's chest should rise smoothly, with chest and abdomen moving in harmony. We speak of "rocking the boat" when the abdomen rises during inspiration and the upper chest lags behind, a sign of respiratory impairment because of upper airway obstruction, partial muscle paralysis, or pulmonary disease such as emphysema. The next glance should be directed at the larynx, which should be quiescent during breathing. With beginning respiratory insufficiency, the larynx moves downward a little with every inspiration, the so-called tracheal tug. The greater the respiratory impairment, the greater the laryngeal excursions with breathing, culminating in the agonal breathing pattern where larynx, floor of mouth, and tongue move with every desperate inspiration. Particularly in children, flaring nostrils indicate respiratory weakness, often enough leading to respiratory failure when small children can no longer muster the effort to overcome weakness or obstruction.

The eyes

Don't forget to check the pupils. When the patient lies face-down or the surgeon works in the face, we must tape the eyes shut to guard against corneal abrasions. At other times, a look at the eyes can be helpful. During general anesthesia, the eyes should be still, the pupils constricted – or at least not dilated – and left should equal right. Light reflexes disappear under surgical anesthesia. Widely dilated pupils – if not the result of mydriatic drugs – indicate grave danger (the "open window to eternity"). The sclera may be injected under light anesthesia as is also true for sleep. And while you are at it, look at the palpebral conjunctiva of the lower lid. The conjunctiva should be pink (not pale with anemia or bluish with hypoxemia or engorged with venous obstruction).

Head lift test

At the end of an anesthetic in which muscle relaxants were used, we need to make sure that the patient has the muscle power to maintain normal ventilation. While the nerve stimulator (see below) is helpful, a simple clinical test is even better: ask the patient to lift his head off the pillow and keep it up for 5 seconds. If he can do that, you can be reasonably assured that he will be able to maintain normal ventilation. When the operative site (neck, upper chest) makes that impossible, we must assess not only the response to the nerve stimulator but also the pattern of breathing and SpO_2.

Auscultation

Cool clinicians wear a stethoscope slung around their necks. Even cooler clinicians actually use the instrument to listen, for example, over the upper trachea: is air escaping at the end of mechanical inspiration? We welcome this sign in small children in whom we avoid compression of the tracheal mucosa with uncuffed endotracheal tubes. In adults we like to inflate the cuff of the endotracheal tube so that a little gas will escape only when we exceed by a few cm H_2O the chosen peak inspiratory pressure. That has two advantages. For one, it assures us that the cuff is not compressing the delicate, tracheal ciliated mucous membrane more than necessary. For another, it provides an emergency escape valve should excessive pressure build up in the breathing circuit. That is rare but has occurred when safety relief valves had failed.

After intubation of the trachea, we listen over both lung fields for breath sounds and check the epigastrium to make sure that we are not delivering gas into the stomach during manual inspiration.

The lowly stethoscope (cheap, non-electronic, sturdy, time honored) often makes the diagnosis for us. No electronic instrument identifies a pneumothorax, but breath sounds on one side and not the other, and the chest rising more on one side than the other spells pneumothorax or endobronchial intubation. Also, consider a patient who becomes tachycardic, hypoxemic, and hypotensive, and assume that pneumothorax ranks high on your list of differential diagnoses. If breath sounds over the left chest equal those over the right and both sides of the chest move equally, a significant pneumothorax moves to the bottom of the differential diagnosis, and pulmonary embolism or cardiac tamponade move up. Don't abandon the stethoscope.

Remember to listen to heart sounds, either through the chest wall or from behind with an esophageal stethoscope. With cardiovascular depression from deep anesthesia, the sounds become muffled. Cardiac tamponade will do the same. In either case, blood pressure will be low and heart rate high. Air embolism may cause the infamous mill wheel murmur produced by blood being beaten into foam in the heart. That is a late sign of air embolism, usually too late to be helpful. Therefore, when worried about the possibility of air embolism, we watch the end-tidal CO_2 (it decreases with pulmonary embolism), and we monitor for air with a precordial Doppler instrument or with a transesophageal echocardiograph. A pulmonary artery catheter will also show signs of increased PA pressure when air bubbles impede blood flow through pulmonary artery branches.

Palpation

How old-fashioned can you get? Putting a hand on the patient will give you all sorts of information. More than just the presence of a pulse, we may assess its quality. Is the patient warm or cold and clammy? (The latter with sympathetic activity causing vasoconstriction and sweating.) Are his muscles fasciculating? (With shivering or after the administration of succinylcholine.) Put the palms of your hands on the clavicles, letting your fingers rest on the upper chest. Does the upper chest rise during spontaneous inspiration? (See above for "rocking the boat".) What is the muscle tone? In spontaneously breathing infants, the intercostal spaces should not retract during inspiration. Infants will also have flaccid fingers with muscle paralysis or deep anesthesia.

Instruments that supplement clinical monitoring

As we begin to focus on instruments to aid us in our monitoring task, we also need to ask for justification for their use. Does this monitor offer benefits that justify the cost (amortization of the instrument and cost of consumable supplies and, don't forget, time needed for application) and the potential hazards inherent with the use of the monitor? Several instruments have been identified as essential minimal monitors *always* to be used. With others, the clinician must decide whether a cost–benefit assessment justifies its use. Many monitors will be used routinely, others only with special indications. We must also point out that, over time, clinical practice changes with changing assessment of the value of this or that monitor.

The American Society of Anesthesiologists has published Minimal Monitoring Standards for patients undergoing general anesthesia.[1] In brief, these standards call for the monitoring of the patient's oxygenation (inspired gas and saturation of arterial blood (SpO_2)), ventilation (capnography and clinical assessment), circulation (ECG, arterial blood pressure), and temperature (a thermometer).

Non-invasive instruments

Some instruments put numbers on observations (feel a thready pulse and assume arterial hypotension; take a blood pressure and put numbers on the hypotension). Others provide information that our senses fail to detect (ECG and capnography, for example).

Blood pressure

The reference point for blood pressure recordings is the heart. For example, when upright, your blood pressure just above the ankle will be much higher than in your upper arm – by the weight of the column of blood between ankle and heart. Conversely, if you worry about cerebral perfusion pressure, remember that the pressure in the upper arm will be higher than that in the head if the patient stands or sits upright. Thus, in a horizontal and recumbent patient, you can monitor blood pressure in the upper or lower arm or just above the ankle (the best place if you have to use the lower extremity) and obtain reasonably accurate readings as long as the cuff is at the level of the heart.

You should be able to take a blood pressure by cuff and stethoscope listening for the Korotkoff sounds. You can also feel a pulse distal to the cuff and register systolic pressure when the distal pulse disappears. Instead of feeling the pulse, you can use a pulse oximeter, which depends on a pulsatile signal to work. Use it while inflating the cuff rather than during deflation. The pulse oximeter averages incoming data and thus takes a little time before reporting a signal, but it stops working rapidly when suddenly deprived of a pulsatile signal, as happens during inflation of the cuff.

The world (at least the Western world) has now taken to oscillometric sphyg-momanometry. The concept is fairly simple. The unit inflates a cuff around the arm (or just above the ankle) and monitors the pressure in the cuff. Well above systolic pressure, the tight cuff transmits no pulsations to the unit. However, as the cuff pressure approaches systolic pressure, the pulsations of the artery begin to cause some oscillation of pressure in the cuff. When the cuff pressure falls just below systolic, the oscillations gain in amplitude, and the clever unit registers systolic pressure. Soon the cuff pressure drops to mean arterial pressure, at which point the oscillations reach their peak amplitude, and the unit recognizes and reports mean arterial pressure. You can imagine that now the oscillations become smaller and smaller and eventually disappear altogether as the cuff pressure drops to and below diastolic pressure. Identifying diastolic pressure presents the algorithm in the unit with the greatest challenge; hence diastolic pressures are more likely to be inaccurate, mean arterial pressure most likely to be accurate, and systolic pressure reasonably accurate. Oscillometric blood pressure recordings have become generally adopted in anesthesia where accuracy within +/− 10% is clinically quite acceptable. Oscillometric measurements may become unreliable when arrhythmias or extremely slow heart rates fool the algorithms that govern the systems.

Pulse oximetry

An old saying goes: *The lack of oxygen not only stops the machinery, it wrecks it.* Hypoxia of the brain first causes confusion, then coma, and eventually irreversible brain damage. Other organs follow that pattern, even though most can survive hypoxia longer than the brain. Thus, knowing whether arterial blood carries oxygen to the organs assumes great importance. Because oxyhemoglobin is red and reduced hemoglobin bluish, this color difference can be exploited to assess the oxygenation of blood. Clinically, we recognize cyanosis, but we cannot well grade the degree of bluishness.

Enter pulse oximetry. The concept is what you might call "elegant." A probe sends light impulses into a finger (or earlobe or nose or toe) and then collects the light that has passed through the tissue. The light comprises two wavelengths: one (infra-red) more likely to be absorbed by oxyhemoglobin, the other (red) by reduced hemoglobin. By rapidly (too rapid for the eye to recognize) alternating the two wavelengths with no light at all, the unit is able to estimate the proportion of oxyhemoglobin to reduced hemoglobin. This is called "functional saturation." Some instruments estimate (*not* measure) the other species of hemoglobin in blood (methemoglobin, carboxyhemoglobin) and compare the oxyhemoglobin as a percentage of the sum of all known hemoglobins. This is called "fractional saturation," which will be a little lower than functional saturation.

We want to know the percentage of oxyhemoglobin saturation in arterial blood (rather than in the tissue or in arterial plus venous blood), therefore we need to catch the saturation reading in the artery, rather than in the whole finger. To accomplish this, the unit functions as a plethysmograph assessing the thickness of the finger (or earlobe or nose or toe). Because the tissue swells a little with each arterial pulsation, the unit can discard data arising during diastole and report on data only recorded during systole, which represent arterial blood. The saturation is reported as SpO_2, the **p** referring to the fact that the measurement is based on pulse oximetry rather than on a direct *in vitro* measurement of oxygen saturation from an **a**rterial blood sample, which would be SaO_2. A healthy person breathing room air at sea level (at least not at Mount Everest) should have an SpO_2 of about 98% $+/- 2\%$. Here is a rough correlation of SpO_2 to arterial partial pressure of oxygen (PaO_2):

SpO_2	PaO_2
100%	100 mmHg or higher
90%	60 mmHg
60%	30 mmHg

In patients with normal lungs and nothing more than a small physiologic shunt (2% to 4%), the PaO_2 should be within spitting range of inspired oxygen pressure. If it is substantially different, a shunt is likely to exist.

There is more to pulse oximetry than outlined here. But we will not dwell on issues of other dyes interfering with the measurements, on the amount of pulsation required, on the influence of venous pulsation, or on the confounding effects of external light. For all of these issues, we refer you to one of many exhaustive texts on monitoring or pulse oximetry.

The electrocardiogram
Intraoperative electrocardiography does not draw on the full power of this sophisticated monitor. Instead of 12 leads, we usually settle for just three or five leads. A little ditty helps with remembering where to put the leads:

White on right, red to ribs, and what is left over to the left shoulder.

With five leads, we add a brown lead for the V 5 position (over the fifth rib in the anterior axillary line) and a green lead that goes to the right side and serves as a ground.

The ECG leads can either be positive or negative, and the lead selector switch changes the polarity of the leads. Think of the negative lead as the exploring sensor.

Lead I looks across the chest:
  White on right shoulder is negative
  Black on left shoulder is positive
  Red on ribs is ground.
Lead II looks along the axis of the heart:
  White on right shoulder is negative
  Black on left shoulder is ground
  Red on ribs is positive.

With the five-lead ECG, lead V5 serves as the exploring, negative electrode overlying the left ventricle; the others (both shoulders and right side) become background.

Many ECG monitors for the operating room offer a "monitoring mode," which is heavily filtered in order to reduce the distortions produced by artifacts induced by motion or electrical noise, e.g., the infamous electrocautery system. While the monitoring mode usually provides clean and stable tracings, the filtering can obscure diagnostic changes or it can mimic changes that will not be seen in a diagnostic 12-lead ECG. Thus, when detecting ST segment depression in the ECG in the monitoring mode, consider the clinical context and switch to diagnostic mode for confirmation before treating the patient. Similarly, when anesthetizing a patient at high risk for myocardial ischemia, use diagnostic mode at least intermittently to evaluate the ST-segment trends.

In the operating room, we are primarily concerned with rhythm and ST segment elevation (impending infarct?) or depression (ischemia?). The best leads to detect such changes are leads II and V5. Lead II shows the best P waves and thus enables us to observe the cardiac rhythm, such as the nodal rhythm frequently observed in the anesthetized patient. Cardiac output and arterial pressure fall a little when the ventricle is deprived of the "atrial kick." Lead V5 looks at the left ventricle, the part of the myocardium most likely to suffer ischemia.

In healthy patients, the information about SpO_2, arterial pressure, and heart rate are more helpful than ECG data. The ECG earns its keep in patients with heart disease and in the rare event of a cardiac arrest and resuscitation. When premature ventricular contractions arise in a patient who did not have them before, we are alerted and begin to search for an explanation. Hypercarbia is a common culprit. Think of ventricular hypoxia when ST segments begin to change (>1.5 mm ST depression or elevation; most ominous is a downward sloping, depressed ST segment), T waves flip, and particularly when the rhythm switches to ventricular tachycardia.

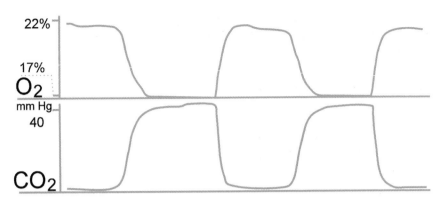

Fig. 7.1 Tracings from a gas monitor that show oxygen (top) and carbon dioxide (bottom) concentrations collected close to the mouth of a healthy volunteer breathing room air. As the person exhales, the oxygen concentration falls while carbon dioxide appears in the collected gas. During inhalation the oxygen analyzer registers room air (about 21% oxygen and no detectable carbon dioxide).

Monitoring respired gases

Capnography

The delivery of carbon dioxide to the lungs depends first on the metabolic production of carbon dioxide. Capnography, therefore, says something about metabolism which may be depressed by cold or fired up during hyperthermia. Capnography depends on blood flow to the lungs. It therefore says something about circulation, specifically that regarding pulmonary blood flow. The delivery of carbon dioxide in the expired gas requires ventilation of alveoli and transport of alveolar gas to the outside. Capnography therefore says something about ventilation. Because the ambient air is free of carbon dioxide (well, not completely free with only about 0.03% in air), the appearance of carbon dioxide in the inspired gas must mean that carbon dioxide is being added to the gas or that the patient is re-inhaling the carbon dioxide he just exhaled, for example from a breathing circuit with a defective valve that causes the dead space in the circuit to increase. Thus, capnography, the measurement of carbon dioxide in the respired gas, really offers rich information that is relatively easily acquired.

The respired gases can be sampled for analysis by aspirating gas from the breathing circuit or from the nose – should the patient be breathing spontaneously – and then delivering it to an analyzer. This is called "side-stream" sampling. We can also clamp an analyzing cuvette directly on the breathing tube so that all the respired gas passes through a system measuring the carbon dioxide, the so-called "on-airway" or "main stream" capnogram.

There are several methods that enable us to measure carbon dioxide. Clinically most often used are infra-red spectroscopy and chemical analysis. Because the infra-red method responds rapidly, it is possible to generate a tracing of the changing carbon dioxide concentration in the respired gases. A capnogram results (Fig. 7.1).

The chemical method is slow but can record approximate ranges of carbon dioxide in gas, which is good enough if you are only interested whether CO_2 is

Fig. 7.2 Volume-based
capnogram. Area *Z* (its top line is
at the level % CO_2 in arterial
blood) represents the deadspace volume of the airway (V_D).
Its right border is obtained by
drawing a vertical line so that
areas *p* and *q* are equal. X plus *p*
represents the volume of
exhaled carbon dioxide. *Y*
represents wasted ventilation
from alveolar deadspace.

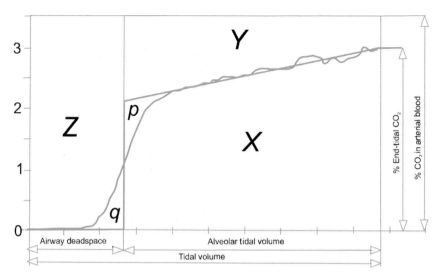

present, for example after intubating the trachea (instead of the esophagus) in an emergency.

One clever method, the volume-based capnogram, plots carbon dioxide over the volume of gas exhaled (Fig. 7.2). It not only lets us estimate the end-tidal concentration of carbon dioxide but it also provides an estimate of deadspace.

Oxygen

When we connect a patient to an atmosphere other than room air, we assume full responsibility for the patient's oxygen supply. The patient might require only 21% oxygen at ambient pressure at sea level, or he might need much more, depending on clinical circumstances. Uncounted patients have died because that seemingly simple requirement was not met either because gases were mixed such that less than 21% oxygen was present in the inspired gas or because a gas other than oxygen came out of the cylinder or pipeline as happens when cylinders are misfilled or pipes delivering gases are switched by mistake. Monitoring oxygen in the inspired gas, therefore, has become mandatory when patients depend on us to prepare their respired gases.

Several methods are available. Ideally, we would like to have a rapidly respond-ing analyzer that generates "oxygrams" as shown in Fig. 7.1. The technology for that relies on mass spectrometry or paramagnetic devices. Many current anes-thesia machines incorporate a fairly slowly responding fuel cell. However, even an instrument with a response time of many seconds suffices.

Anesthetic gases

With side-stream gas monitors, it becomes possible to use the technology incorporated into capnography to analyze nitrous oxide and the halogenated inhalation anesthetics. The response time of these analyzers enables us to monitor both inspired and expired gas concentrations. We can thus watch what concentration the patient inhales. This frequently differs from the concentration set at the vaporizer which delivers gas to the breathing circuit where the fresh gases are diluted by the gases the patient re-inhales (see Anesthesia machine chapter).

Temperature

The body of an adult patient can absorb many calories before becoming noticeably warmer or, conversely, will cool only relatively slowly when losing heat by radiation (which accounts for most of the heat loss), evaporation (next in importance), convection, and conduction (least important).[2] However, monitoring the temperature, regardless how slowly it changes, becomes important in babies and small children and in patients exposed to large heat losses as occur with lengthy intraabdominal or intrathoracic operations. In patients whose temperature drifts down to 35 °C, wound infections may be more common. Other side effects of hypothermia include reduced enzyme activity and shivering (which increases oxygen consumption potentially contributing to myocardial ischemia), as well as the patient's discomfort.

Central blood in the vena cava or pulmonary artery gives the most representative "core temperature." Tympanic membrane, esophagus, under the tongue, and the rectum offer other sites. During endotracheal anesthesia, esophageal temperatures can be measured easily with the help of an esophageal stethoscope that carries a temperature probe (thermistor) at its tip.

Skin temperatures can be measured in the axilla and on the forehead. For the latter site, temperature sensing adhesives are available that change their color with changing temperatures. Their accuracy is limited not only by the fact that ambient temperatures affect skin temperature but also because the temperature-sensitive liquid crystals do not offer good resolution.

Neuromuscular function

Because we use neuromuscular blocking agents (muscle relaxants, for short) so frequently, we need to monitor the degree of relaxation. Clinical judgment goes a long way, but instruments can gauge the degree of relaxation and provide numerical assessment. For this purpose, we use a nerve stimulator that delivers short pulses of a direct current. We use two stick-on electrodes placed fairly close together (Fig. 7.3) over the course of a nerve (usually the ulnar nerve close to the wrist), and select one of several patterns of stimuli. Ideally, the current is well below the level to stimulate the muscle directly, as a healthy muscle will respond to strong, direct stimulation even in the presence of neuromuscular blocking agents. Thus, we are looking for maximal stimulation of the nerve only. Submaximal stimulation of the nerve can induce variability of response and thus make it

Table 7.2. Neuromuscular blockade monitor pattern descriptions

	Frequency	Pattern	Comments
Train of four	2 Hz	Four twitches 0.5 s apart	Repeats every 12 seconds
Tetanus	50 to 100 Hz	For 5 seconds	
Post-tetanic stimulation	Single stimulus at 1 Hz		Follows a 5 second tetanus
Double burst	2 Hz	Three twitches, a 750 ms pause, followed by two more twitches	

Fig. 7.3 Neuromuscular
blockade (twitch) monitoring.
Electrodes placed over the
course of the ulnar nerve.

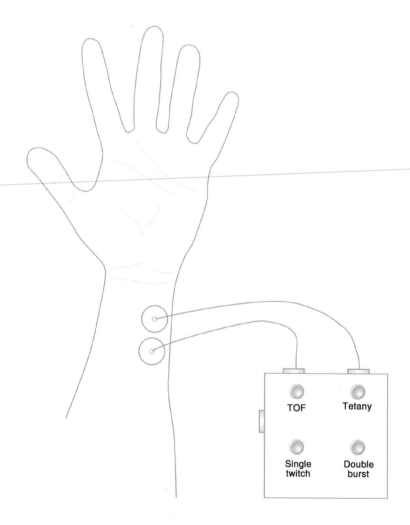

Supramaximal nerve stimulation responses during depolarizing and non-depolarizing block

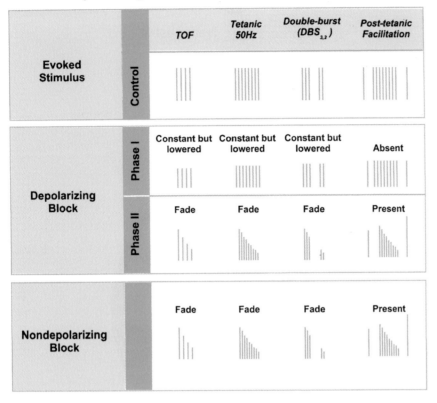

		TOF	Tetanic 50Hz	Double-burst (DBS$_{3,2}$)	Post-tetanic Facilitation
Evoked Stimulus	Control				
Depolarizing Block	Phase I	Constant but lowered	Constant but lowered	Constant but lowered	Absent
	Phase II	Fade	Fade	Fade	Present
Nondepolarizing Block		Fade	Fade	Fade	Present

Fig. 7.4 Neuromuscular blockade monitor patterns. The figure shows the response we expect to see in a normal muscle before giving any muscle relaxants (control), after the administration of succinylcholine (Phase I), a depolarizing muscle relaxant which, after continued administration, assumes the pattern of a so-called Phase II block, and finally following the administration of a non-depolarizing muscle relaxant, resulting in a pattern resembling the Phase II block from succinylcholine (Reproduced with permission from Kalli, I. S. in Kirby *et al.* *Clinical Anesthesia Practice*, W. B. Saunders, p. 446, 2002.)

impossible to tell whether an observed depression must be attributed to neuro-muscular blockade or inadequate stimulation.

The most commonly used patterns of stimulation are shown in Table 7.2, with the typical patterns of response depicted in Fig. 7.4. In addition to the response to nerve stimulation, we like to check the patient's muscle power if possible. Full return of muscle power can be assumed if the patient can lift his head off the pillow for 5 seconds, or bite on a tongue depressor so that you cannot withdraw it. If we suspect residual neuromuscular blockade in the PACU, we ask if the patient has double vision or difficulty sitting up or swallowing.

Doppler and ultrasound

The Doppler principle has been applied to monitoring in anesthesia. We can place a Doppler pencil probe over a vessel to identify blood flow or, with a broader emitter/receiver head, place it over the chest to detect the blood flow in the right

Fig. 7.5 Transesophageal
echocardiography (TEE).
Standard planes through the
heart. The probe is positioned for
the transgastric view. By moving
it we obtain the other two views.

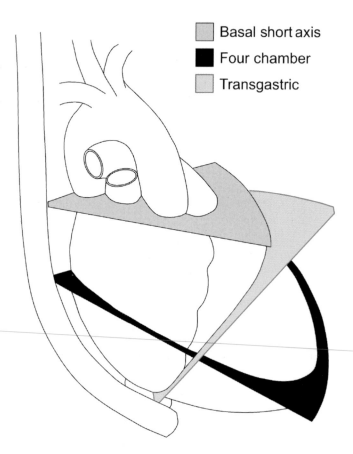

■ Basal short axis
■ Four chamber
■ Transgastric

atrium. When air appears in the blood flowing into the heart, it changes the
reflective characteristics of the blood, easily detected by the Doppler signal, which
is transformed into a swooshing noise.

While ultrasound has been used for many years to spy on babies still in the
womb and to view the functioning heart through the chest wall, more recently the
equipment has been miniaturized into a finger-sized probe that views the heart
from behind, through the wall of the esophagus (Fig. 7.5). This advance gives us
a hands-free, relatively stable (and relatively non-invasive) view of the heart that
does not impinge on the operative field. The technology continues to advance but
currently allows views from multiple angles and Doppler analysis of flow through
the valves and even the coronaries (for the experienced ultrasonographer). While
invasive pressure monitoring can give indirect insights into cardiac physiology,
with TEE we can actually *see* the heart doing its work. We can assess preload
(how full is the ventricle?), contractility (how much are the walls thickening?),
and ischemia (are there sections of the ventricular walls that lag behind?). During

cardiac surgery, we can evaluate valve repairs and ASD closures. TEE is also a great way to detect air emboli.

This is probably the shortest description of a subject that has spawned uncounted papers, chapters, and books with exhaustive explanations. Studying them will introduce the reader to the complexities of the subject, but fairly intensive practice will be required to become facile with this promising monitoring modality.

The electroencephalogram and evoked responses

In anesthesia, we expend much more effort in monitoring the cardiovascular and respiratory system than the nervous system, even though anesthesia is all about putting nervous function out of commission long enough to abolish awareness or at least the perception of pain. The reason for our bias against monitoring nervous activities is that we can afford to overdose the nervous functions and put them completely to rest as long as we continue to satisfy the basal needs for substrate and oxygen to brain and nerves. Hence, we worry more about the circulation than about the brain. However, when the systemic circulation is doing well but blood supply to all or parts of the brain or spinal cord is threatened, we need to monitor their function. Two methods are available: the electroencephalogram and evoked responses.

The EEG as recorded by experts requires a montage with many electrodes. In anesthesia, that is not practical and in the operating room, you will rarely see more than a couple of leads plus a ground. The typical EEG of an awake individual shows rapid fire wiggles of low amplitude. With increasing depression of the central nervous system, the frequency of the wiggles decreases, and the amplitude increases. Before the EEG becomes flat, showing no electrical activity, it goes through a stage of burst suppression in which brief electrical activity alternates with longer periods of electrical silence. Figure 7.6 shows these typical patterns which can be described by the frequency of their waves and the amplitude of their excursions.

The EEG can be processed to make interpretation more convenient. Several methods have been published. A commercial success has been the BIS (Bispectral index) monitor, which translates an automatic analysis of the EEG waveforms (obtained from forehead leads) into a unit-less number between 0 and 100 – the higher the number, the more awake the patient. In general, a BIS of 60 or less is associated – most of the time – with general anesthesia. However, even in physiologic (not pharmacologic) sleep, the BIS can dip well below 60. Thus, we still need to consider the context (drugs, surgical stimulation) in which we observe BIS values. It will have served us well if it helps us to avoid excessively deep anesthesia – which might be harmful – and all too light anesthesia – which carries the risk of intraoperative awareness. Anesthesia that is neither

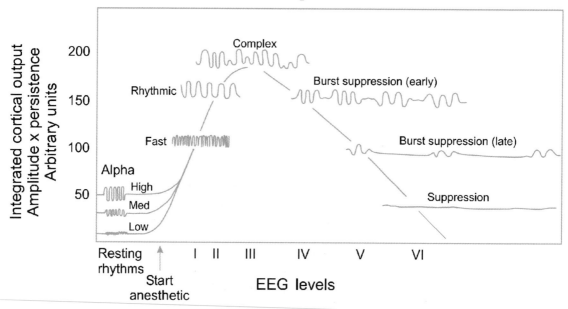

Diagram of average pattern changes during anesthesia

Fig. 7.6 Electroencephalogram patterns with anesthesia. Changes in the electroencephalogram are shown with increasing depths of anesthesia. Note that the alpha rhythm amplitude range decreases as anesthesia is administered (Martin, J.T., Faulconer, A. and Bickford R.G. Electroencephalography in anesthesiology. *Anesthesiology*, 20:360, 1959, with permission).

too deep nor too light can speed postoperative recovery (wake-up and PACU time).

When we need to monitor the integrity of specific neuronal pathways, we use the evoked potential. Here, we apply a volley of either somatic, auditory, or visual stimuli. The system then automatically scans the EEG, looking for responses to the stimuli and filtering out all other activity in the EEG. It then presents an evoked potential response with characteristic latencies and amplitude of positive and negative deflections. Categorically, we can say that a central response to a peripheral stimulus signifies that the sensory pathways between periphery and brain are conducting impulses and that the brain is capable of responding. If the response is delayed or muted, it is either because the pathways have been affected or the brain is depressed, for example by anesthetics. You can easily imagine that the monitoring of evoked responses can be helpful when the integrity of the pathways are jeopardized by trauma or the surgical intervention, e.g., scoliosis correction.

Invasive monitors

Arterial catheter

The ease with which a small catheter can be inserted into an artery, usually the radial, has caused many patients to be monitored with arterial catheters (often

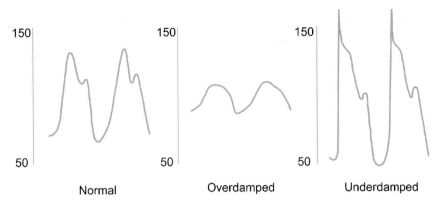

150   150   150

50   50   50

Normal   Overdamped   Underdamped

Fig. 7.7 Arterial pressure waveform patterns. Note the flattened peak of an overdamped waveform, often corrected by removing small bubbles in the pressure tubing and/or flushing the arterial catheter. In an underdamped waveform, an extreme peak introduces error in the systolic and diastolic data.

called "lines" which is not an ideal term, as a line has no lumen, something arterial and venous catheters distinctly possess). Before inserting a catheter into a radial (rarely the ulnar) artery, many clinicians like to check the patency of the volar arterial arch that connects radial and ulnar arteries. In the so-called Allen's test, the hand is blanched, both arteries occluded by external pressure, then one occluded artery is freed. If now the entire hand, rather than the vascular bed of just one artery, turns pink, we accept the idea that the volar arch is patent and should one artery become obstructed by a clot or through damage to the intima, the other artery will prevent necrosis of fingers.

For this and all other invasive pressure measurements, we use saline or heparin-filled non-compressible (pressure) tubing connected to a transducer, which converts the pressure waveform into an electrical signal. We need to make sure that the instrument is properly calibrated and that the zero level (open to air) is at the level of the heart. Two problems can cause the system to report faulty systolic and diastolic – but usually correct mean – pressures. When the signal is damped, for example owing to an air bubble somewhere in the tubing, the systolic pressure will read falsely low, and the diastolic pressure falsely high. When the system is not damped enough, it might ring (like a bouncing spring), now reporting falsely high systolic (and low diastolic) pressures (see Fig. 7.7).

Arterial catheters give ready access to arterial blood and thus to an analysis of blood gases. When drawing arterial blood for analysis, be sure you are not diluting the blood and that you have the analysis performed without delay so that the normal metabolism of the cells does not affect the results.

Central venous catheter

Placement of a central venous catheter offers not only the ability to determine the central venous pressure but also an avenue for rapid infusions (see Vascular access). Because no valve separates the vena cavae from the atrium, central venous pressure (CVP) reflects right atrial pressure. Similarly, when the tricuspid valve is open, and pressure has equalized between the atrium and ventricle

Fig. 7.8 Central venous pressure
waveform. The *a* wave is from
*a*trial contraction, *c* from *c*losure
of the tricuspid valve and
ventricular contraction; *v* from
*v*enous filling of the atrium.

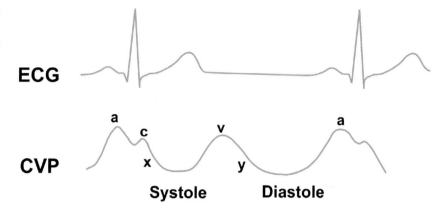

(end-diastole), the CVP will also reflect right ventricular end-diastolic pressure
(RVEDP). If we assume a normal ventricular compliance (pressure–volume relationship), we now have an indication of the end-diastolic volume or preload.
However, because of its intrathoracic location, the central venous catheter also
records pressures in the thorax as a whole, and thus, CVP fluctuates with ventilation. In a spontaneously breathing patient, normal pressures might range from
-2 to $+6$ cm H_2O. If we then mechanically ventilate that patient's lungs, pressures
of $+4$ to $+12$ (or more with high peak inspiratory pressures) can be expected – this
without changing his intravascular volume and, in fact, likely *lowering* his preload
as venous return is hampered by high intrathoracic pressure. The shape of the
CVP waveform reflects the cardiac cycle (Fig. 7.8) and may suggest conditions
that limit the extrapolation of preload from CVP, such as tricuspid valve disease
or a poorly compliant ventricle. As with all monitors, when interpreting CVP data
we must consider the clinical scenario and look more at trends in a given patient
than the actual values.

Pulmonary artery catheter

Once the catheter is properly positioned, best in an area where the balance
between blood flow and ventilation favors flow (below the level of the left atrium
or zone III according to West),[3] the cuff can be inflated, blocking the vessel so that
the tip of the catheter no longer senses PA pressure. Instead, it now looks downstream and registers pressures submitted retrograde from the left atrium. This
pulmonary artery occlusion or wedge pressure helps to identify situations affecting left ventricular preload. However, as with the CVP, many factors can influence
the readings, e.g., mitral valve disease, pulmonary hypertension. Normal data
appear in Table 7.3.

A number of refinements add utility to the PA catheter. For one, a thermistor at
the tip of the catheter can record the temperature of the blood flowing past. After
the injection of cold saline through a port situated in the vena cava, the observed

Table 7.3. Normal pulmonary artery pressure data

Location	mm Hg
Right atrium	3
Right ventricle	25/5
Pulmonary artery	25/10
Pulmonary artery occlusion or wedge pressure	8

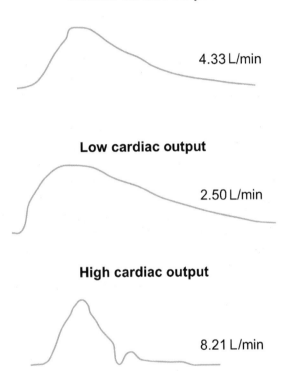

Normal cardiac output

4.33 L/min

Low cardiac output

2.50 L/min

High cardiac output

8.21 L/min

Fig. 7.9 Thermodilution cardiac output curves.

temperature changes at the tip of the catheter make it possible to estimate the cardiac output. When the output is low, blood will flow slowly past the thermistor, and a large thermodilution curve will result. Conversely, with a large cardiac output, the thermodilution curve will be small (Fig. 7.9).

We can also monitor the oxygen saturation of central venous blood either intermittently by drawing samples for the laboratory, or continuously by incorporating an oximeter in the catheter. When oxygen content of arterial blood and oxygen consumption are constant, a drop in venous oxygen saturation indicates a decrease in tissue blood flow, i.e., cardiac output.

Table 7.4. Monitoring in anesthesia

	Qualities measured	Pros	Cons
Cardiac			
Palpation	Pulse rate, rhythm and quality; thrill; point of maximal impulse	Inexpensive, non-invasive	
Auscultation	Rate, rhythm, S3, S4, murmur, air embolism	Inexpensive, non-invasive	
Non-invasive blood pressure	Blood pressure	Non-invasive	May have a problem with arrhythmias
ECG	Rate, rhythm, ischemia	Non-invasive	Non-specific
TEE	Function, volume, ischemia	Few confounding factors	Expensive, requires expertise, uncomfortable for the awake patient
Arterial catheter	Blood pressure, ABG	Beat-to-beat BP, easy access to arterial blood	Invasive
Central venous catheter	Preload	High volume catheter useful for resuscitation	Invasive
Pulmonary artery catheter	Preload, cardiac output, RV and PA pressures, mixed venous oxygen saturation	Gold standard for cardiac output, availability of mixed venous O_2	Invasive, significant rate of potentially severe complications, expensive
Pulmonary			
Auscultation	Breath sounds, pneumothorax	Inexpensive, non-invasive	
Pulse oximetry	Oxyhemoglobin saturation	Inexpensive, non-invasive	Inaccurate with carbon monoxide, severe anemia
Capnography	Inhaled and exhaled carbon dioxide	Gold standard to document tracheal position of ETT	Not quantitative unless intubated
Arterial blood gas	Oxygenation, ventilation, acid–base status	Accurate measure	Invasive, usually not continuous
Neurologic			
Twitch monitor	Neuromuscular blockade	Inexpensive	Insensitive unless at least 70% of receptors blocked
BIS	"Depth of anesthesia"	Non-invasive	Not always a leading indicator of light anesthesia
Evoked potentials	Specific neuronal pathways	Relatively specific for the pathway investigated	Expensive, requires technical expertise for interpretation, affected by many anesthetic agents

PA catheters have come under much criticism because they may not reveal as much as originally hoped for, and they are highly invasive and saddled with a measurable rate of sometimes life-threatening complications including but not limited to dysrhythmias, thrombosis, infection, and devastating pulmonary artery rupture.[4] Much less invasively, transesophageal echocardiography offers a great advantage over the PA catheter. PA catheters generate pressure and flow data; TEE shows volumes and function of all four chambers and valves.

Thus we have many monitors at our disposal (Table 7.4), with new ones arriving regularly. Each has strengths, weaknesses, risks, and potential benefits. No monitor is therapeutic in itself but requires the skill and vigilance of a trained observer to interpret the information in the context of the ever-changing clinical picture.

NOTES

1. http://www.anest.ufl.edu/EA.
2. Radiation: loss of heat to the atmosphere, Evaporation: loss of heat as fluids absorbed from surface (airway, exposed viscous), Convection: loss of heat to a cold air mass moving across the body, Conduction: transfer of heat to a colder object in direct contact (OR table).
3. John B. West (1928–) described ventilation and perfusion inequality in the lung, and wrote a very nice and readable textbook reviewing the concepts. *Respiratory Physiology: The Essentials*. 6th edn, 2000.
4. American Society of Anesthesiologists Task Force on Pulmonary Artery Catheterization (1993). Practice guidelines for pulmonary artery catheterization. *Anesthesiology*, **79**, 380–426.

8

The anesthesia machine

As anesthetic agents and techniques have evolved, so have the delivery systems. Modern anesthesia requires the ability to administer gases and vapors in the desired combinations, often while mechanically ventilating the patient's lungs. Here we present step-by-step the concepts on which anesthesia machines are based. We are starting with systems that sport neither valves nor means to store gases, advance to systems that can store gases – which requires a couple of valves, and advance to systems in which the patient rebreathes his exhaled gas – but without carbon dioxide. Thus, we will have set the stage for the modern anesthesia machine. A nice interactive computerized diagram can be found at http://www.anest.uf/edu/EA.

Systems without gas storage

If we have to give anesthesia on the North Pole, and we have nothing but a can of diethyl ether, we can give a fine anesthetic by dripping the ether on a cloth held over the patient's mouth. That will work also with halothane and isoflurane. Early anesthetists used masks (Fig. 8.1) on which to drape the cloth.

Back from the North Pole, assume we have a patient who weighs 70 kg, has a tidal volume of 600 mL, a respiratory rate of 10 breaths/min and an I : E (inspiratory to expiratory) ratio of 1 to 2; that is, he spends twice as much time exhaling (and pausing between breaths) than inhaling. Assume his trachea to be intubated. All his respired gases flow through the tubing connecting his endotracheal tube to the source of oxygen. (Fig. 8.2). We wish to provide his lungs with 100% oxygen. To achieve this, his exhaled gas needs to be vented through a T near the mouth. This T will also allow him to pull in room air during inspiration, diluting his FiO$_2$. What oxygen flow rate will prevent such entrainment of room air? The easy answer: the oxygen flow rate must match his inspiratory flow rate (which, by the way, is not constant). The total amount of oxygen the system must deliver then will equal his minute ventilation of 6000 mL, but this volume must be given over only 1/3 of a minute (with an I : E of 1:2). The technology for such an arrangement, i.e.,

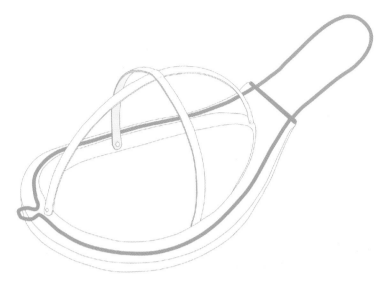

Fig. 8.1 A Schimmelbusch mask; used to keep gauze off the patient's face while administering open drop ether anesthesia. (Named for Curt Schimmelbusch (1860–1895), a German surgeon.)

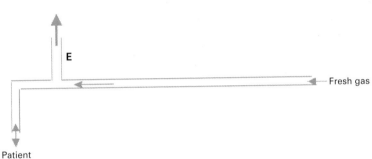

Fig. 8.2 The simplest arrangement of delivering gas to the patient. Fresh gas flows throughout the respiratory cycle. If its flow matches the patient's inspiratory gas flow, the patient will not inhale room air through the T of the expiratory limb (E); however, the fresh gas flowing throughout exhalation will be lost to the outside.

to flow oxygen only during inspiration, exists in ICU ventilators. In anesthesia machines, we instead have continuous gas flow throughout the respiratory cycle. In the example above, during exhalation, the continuing oxygen flow has nowhere to go but to escape, together with the patient's exhaled gas, to the outside. We still must meet his inspiratory flow demand, delivering his minute volume during inspiration (in 1/3 minute), and we would lose all of the oxygen (2/3 of the total) flowing during expiration. Thus, using this simple system in a patient with an I : E ratio of 1:2, we would need a fresh gas flow three times as large as his minute volume.

Single-valve system with gas storage

In order to save gas, we can provide for storage of the gas. Well known is the Mapleson system,[1] often used during resuscitation and during transport of a

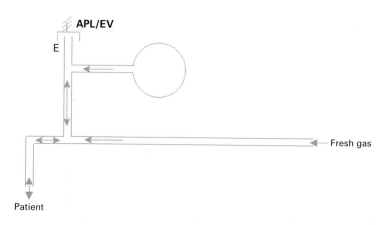

Fig. 8.3 The arrangement of Fig. 8.2 has been expanded to include an adjustable one-way valve (APL: adjustable pressure-limiting; EV: expiratory valve) that, when open, lets the patient exhale to the outside and, when partially closed, enables the anesthesiologist to generate pressure by squeezing the bag and thus inflating the patient's lungs while spilling some gas to the outside. Depending on the fresh gas flow, more or less of the patient's carbon dioxide will be vented to the outside. In other words, with inadequate fresh gas flow, the patient will re-inhale some or much of his exhaled carbon dioxide. E: expiratory limb.

patient who requires mechanical ventilation. The system shown in Fig. 8.3 is properly called a Mapleson **D** (as there are different arrangements lettered A through F).

Figure 8.4 shows the real thing. It is light and deceptively simple. To prevent rebreathing of exhaled carbon dioxide requires a relatively high fresh gas flow, both to meet inspiratory demand and to wash exhaled CO_2 out of the tubing. Here, the excess gas escapes through an adjustable one-way (pop-off) valve that prevents entrainment of room air. The pressure required to open the spring-loaded valve can be varied, enabling us to generate enough pressure (by squeezing the bag) to inflate the patient's lungs. Slow respiratory rates help because, during a long pause between inspirations, the fresh gas will push the exhaled gas toward the pop-off valve. During spontaneous ventilation, the fresh gas flow should be as high as 200 to 300 mL/kg; for our patient, that would be 14–21 L/min. With manually controlled ventilation, 100 to 200 mL/kg will do. We will occasionally observe lower flow rates in clinical usage, causing unintended rebreathing of carbon dioxide. To be sure, err on the high side – which wastes a little gas and has no disadvantage

Fig. 8.4 Line drawing of a Mapleson System. The Mapleson (D) system finds extensive use in anesthesia. While simple, the system requires a source of compressed oxygen. See text.

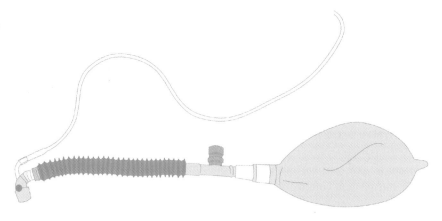

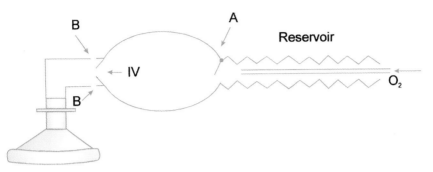

Fig. 8.5 The self-inflating bag. Conceptual diagram of a self-inflating resuscitation bag that prevents rebreathing of exhaled gas but enables the clinician to ventilate the patient's lungs either with room air or with oxygen delivered into a reservoir. B denotes the exhalation ports, which become occluded during inspiration when the inspiratory valve (IV) opens. The one-way valve, "A," closes when the bag is squeezed, forcing gas toward the facemask during inspiration. The valve opens as the bag re-expands, allowing oxygen-rich reservoir gas to fill the breathing bag (if using the system without an oxygen source, the reservoir gas will consist of room air).

to the patient – rather than on the low side, which causes rebreathing of carbon dioxide, the very problem patients in respiratory distress should be spared.

The Mapleson systems require compressed gas.

Multi-valve system with gas storage

A self-inflating bag provides an alternative that enables the resuscitator to ventilate the patient's lungs with room air or, if oxygen is available, with air enriched with oxygen. For the latter to succeed, the self-inflating bag must have a reservoir in which oxygen can accumulate during inspiration (see Fig. 8.5).

Without a self-inflating bag, gas has to be admitted to the breathing system under pressure. Figure 8.6 shows a simple arrangement. We incorporate a bag and two valves. Now the fresh gas accumulates in the bag during exhalation when the inspiratory valve closes and the expiratory valve opens (venting CO_2-laden gas to the atmosphere). During inspiration the valves swap roles: the inspiratory valve opens and the expiratory one closes. Such valves have little resistance, perhaps 1 or 2 cm H_2O, and thus will easily open during the respiratory cycle. This works for a patient breathing spontaneously. Again, an adjustable pressure-limiting valve on top of the expiratory limb enables us to ventilate the patient's lungs.

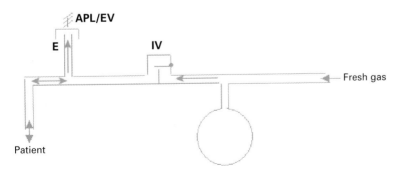

Fig. 8.6 After adding another one-way valve and moving the bag, we arrive at a system that reduces the required fresh gas flow to that of the patient's minute ventilation. During exhalation, the inspiratory valve (IV) closes, enabling the continuously flowing fresh gas to accumulate in the breathing bag. E: expiratory limb; APL: adjustable pressure-limiting valve; EV: expiratory valve.

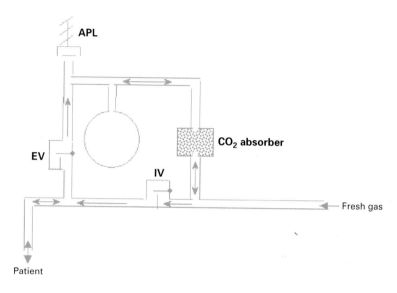

Fig. 8.7 A circle system has been formed by tapping into the expiratory limb to attach the reservoir bag so that it can collect exhaled gas. During inspiration, the gas will now be drawn out of the reservoir bag, pass through the carbon dioxide absorber, and then join the fresh gas. For abbreviations see Fig. 8.6.

Systems with carbon dioxide absorption

In anesthesia, because of the cost (and ozone-depleting qualities) of volatile anesthetic agents, we prefer to conserve even more gas. Furthermore, the patient does not consume all inhaled oxygen (at rest, a patient consumes only a small portion of the inhaled oxygen, reducing the FiO_2 of 0.21 to an FeO_2 of 0.17). Thus, we save a lot if we have to do nothing more than replace the oxygen the patient consumes (for the average adult at rest – about 250 to 300 mL/min). We need to remove the carbon dioxide, of which our resting patient generates about as much (depending on his respiratory quotient) as he consumes oxygen. Figure 8.7 shows the arrangement. We simply formed a circle (conceptually, if not diagrammatically) by connecting the expiratory and inspiratory limbs. The two valves in the circle assure a one-way flow of gases in the circuit. We still have the APL valve and the breathing bag, but we have incorporated a carbon dioxide absorber. Now we can reduce the inflow of oxygen (and anesthetic gases) into the circle quite drastically.

With this circle system, we have the basic anesthesia machine. Now, all we need to add are flow meters for other gases (nitrous oxide, air) and vaporizers that let us introduce anesthetic vapor to the fresh gas flowing into the breathing system. We also have the option of switching on a mechanical ventilator.

Using a handy diagram of a modern anesthesia machine (Fig. 8.8), we point out several features. The system receives compressed gases from the hospital's gas supply; it has a back-up gas supply stored in cylinders; it reduces the high pressure in the cylinders to manageable levels in the machine; it has adjustable vaporizers for halogenated anesthetics (isoflurane, desflurane and sevoflurane – but

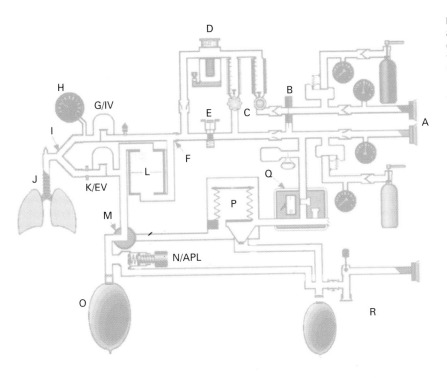

Fig. 8.8 Diagram of a traditional anesthesia machine. To bring the computer animation to life and for explanation and operating instruction, please check: http://www.anest.ufl.edu/EA. A: The gases enter the anesthesia machine either from hospital piping or from cylinders attached to the anesthesia machine; B: the so-called fail-safe system that stops the flow of nitrous oxide should the pressure in the oxygen pipe drop; C: the flowmeters with which to set the flow rates for gases – here only oxygen and nitrous oxide. On many machines, there will be a flow meter for air and sometimes one for helium; D: the vaporizer. Many machines carry more than one vaporizer but they are always arranged so that we can use only one at a time; E: the oxygen flush button, which admits a high flow of oxygen under pressure to the system. If pressed during the ventilator's inspiratory phase, excessive pressure can build up in the breathing system with the potential of causing barotrauma to the patient's lungs; F: fresh gas inlet to the breathing circuit; G/IV: the inspiratory one-way valve; H: manometer registering the pressure in the breathing circuit; I: the "Y" piece, named after its shape. It connects the breathing circle to the patient; J: trachea and lungs of the patient; K/EV: the expiratory one-way valve. As long as this and the inspiratory valve function properly, the breathing circle imposes no significant apparatus dead space, extending only into the "Y" piece; L: the carbon dioxide absorber; M: the selector valve, which funnels the gas either into the breathing bag – as shown here – or to the ventilator; N/APL: the "pop-off" or APL (adjustable pressure limiting) valve enables gas to escape when the pressure in the breathing circuit exceeds a selected value; O: the breathing bag; P: ventilator bellows; Q: ventilator controls; R: scavenging system.

permits only one agent to be administered at a time); and it funnels the anesthetic-laden fresh gas into the breathing circuit that has a carbon dioxide absorber. The system makes it possible for the patient to breathe spontaneously into a breathing bag, which can be manually compressed if necessary, to ventilate the patient's lungs. While all systems have mechanical ventilators, the design of these differs markedly among manufacturers of anesthesia machines.

The hospital system also provides suction that removes waste gases. Such scavenging keeps the air in the operating room virtually free of anesthetic agents presumed to present a hazard to personnel, particularly pregnant women.

Modern anesthesia machines have a bevy of safety features:

- All gas hoses have connectors specific to the gas. This makes a mix-up of gases unlikely. It does not guarantee that oxygen comes out of the oxygen pipeline should the pipes have been switched during construction or repairs, an occurrence not all that rare.
- One-way valves prevent gas from flowing from the cylinders into the anesthesia machine as long as the system is connected to the pipeline. The pipeline pressure exceeds the reduced cylinder pressure. This arrangement prevents drainage of the cylinders while the machine is connected to wall supply. This also means that one has to disconnect the machine from the wall should it become necessary to use gas from the cylinders.

- A safety valve closes the flow of nitrous oxide should the pressure in the oxygen conduit drop below a critical level. This so-called *fail-safe valve* makes it impossible to give nitrous oxide without pressure in the oxygen conduits.
- A back-up to the fail-safe valve is the linkage between nitrous oxide and oxygen, which prevents the delivery of less than 25% oxygen.
- The gases in the breathing system are monitored and their concentration displayed.

The machine depicted diagrammatically in Fig. 8.8 can be brought to life by signing on to the Internet under http://www.anest.ufl.edu/EA. There we can manipulate controls, operate the ventilator, and watch the flow of color-coded gases. We can even cause the system to have faults and observe the consequences. With the animated diagrams comes a workbook that will not only explain features of the machine but also offer self-tests.

Anesthesia breathing circuits have come a long way since the open-drop ether days; however, with increased sophistication also comes a need for heightened awareness. These systems, if improperly used, e.g., inadequate fresh gas flow, inappropriately tightened APL valve, faulty expiratory valve, incorrect setting of the ventilator, undiscovered disconnection, can and do cause significant injury. Because of these many potential dangers, we monitor gas flows, pressures in the breathing circle, tidal and minute volumes, inspired oxygen, and inhaled and exhaled carbon dioxide. Many of these variables come with alarms that sound at adjustable thresholds.

NOTE

1. His department head at the University of Wales assigned William Wellesley Mapleson (1926–) to study gas flows through five existing breathing systems in 1954. Mapleson was surprised to later hear his name attached to the alphabetic labels he had conjured up.

Part II

Applied physiology and pharmacology

9

Anesthesia and the cardiovascular system

Surgical procedures and anesthesia confront the cardiovascular system with a triple threat: trauma, blood loss, and depressant drugs. Trauma triggers a cascade of hormones; if that were not enough, the surgeon might constrict the vena cava, compress a lung, trigger reflexes, and handle the gut, causing sequestration of fluid in traumatized tissue. Exposed pleural and peritoneal lining lets water evaporate, not to mention blood loss and the potential of small clots. To this onslaught, anesthesia adds depressant drugs, induces ventilation/perfusion mismatches with mechanical ventilation (which turns respiratory mechanics upside-down by imposing positive pressure during inhalation), and then infuses cold solutions that are never quite the same as the real thing. Aware of all of these factors, the anesthesiologist appreciates the stresses imposed on the patient and does his or her best to keep the system as close as possible to "how Mother Nature intended it." To that end, we must have a firm grasp of physiology. Let's start with the most visible outward sign of the cardiovascular system: blood pressure.

Blood pressure and its determinants

To understand how surgery and anesthesia affect blood pressure, we must consider its basic components (Fig. 9.1). First, *afterload*, the combination of all resistances against which the heart must eject. Its aliases include systemic vascular resistance (SVR) and total peripheral resistance (TPR). This parameter cannot be measured, but rather is calculated based on the relationship of pressure to flow:[1]

$$SVR = \frac{(MAP - CVP) \times 80}{CO}$$

where MAP = mean arterial pressure, CVP = central venous pressure, and CO = cardiac output.

The vasomotor center influences the diameter of peripheral vessels through sympathetic α_1 innervation. SVR, then, changes with anything that affects the

Fig. 9.1 Determinants of blood pressure. Each successive level gives its dependent factors (e.g., blood pressure depends on cardiac output and afterload). For all but the parameters in parentheses, the relationship is direct, for example, increasing afterload *increases* blood pressure but *decreases* ejection fraction. Some inter-relationships are identified (e.g., as heart rate increases, it adversely affects filling time (shortened diastole), lowering the LVEDV). The flowchart can be helpful in recognizing the effects of pathologic changes. For example, hemorrhage (decreased intravascular volume on the bottom row, and following the chart toward the top) decreases venous return, LVEDV, stroke volume, cardiac output, and blood pressure. We can improve the blood pressure through any of the independent parameters (shaded): increase afterload (α_1), heart rate (β_1), contractility (also β_1), intravascular volume (best choice), venous pressure gradient (e.g., Trendelenburg's position), and/or *reduce* venous capacity (α_1). In fact, the baroreflex and Starling's Forces start working on all this even before we intervene. LVEDV: left ventricular end-diastolic volume, LVESD: left ventricular end-systolic volume, venous P gradient: venous pressure gradient from distal to proximal – a larger gradient encourages more blood return to the heart.

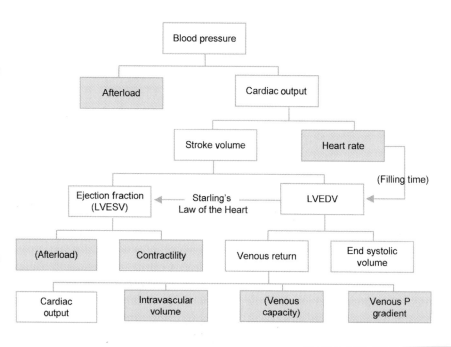

vasomotor center (the baroreflex (see below), anesthetics), the sympathetic chain (neuraxial (epidural or spinal) anesthesia), α_1 receptors (catecholamines, vaso-pressors), or smooth muscle of the vessel wall directly (histamine, anesthetic agents, nitric oxide).

Cardiac output, the other determinant of blood pressure, depends on heart rate and stroke volume. *Heart rate* is somewhat more complex than it may first seem, with both sympathetic (β_1) and parasympathetic innervation "battling it out" for supremacy. Here, the baroreflex exerts its influence, as well as the majority of pharmacologic agents we use to manipulate the heart rate.

For *stroke volume*, there are multiple factors in play, beginning with *Starling's law of the heart*[2] (Fig. 9.2). Basically, it states that the heart tends to pump out all the blood it receives, in essence maintaining the same end-systolic volume. Note the normally sloped Starling curve: stroke volume increases directly with the filling volume (measured as left ventricular end-diastolic pressure (LVEDP), central venous pressure (CVP) or pulmonary capillary wedge pressure (PCWP). Think of the actin and myosin filaments having an optimal overlap. With little ventricular volume, they are completely overlapped and can generate little pressure. Similarly, at some point, they become over-stretched, beyond their optimal overlap, causing a reduction in force, represented by the flat or downward sloping portion at the right-most end of the curve. Notice the flatness of the heart failure curve; increasing preload does not really help these patients. From the Starling

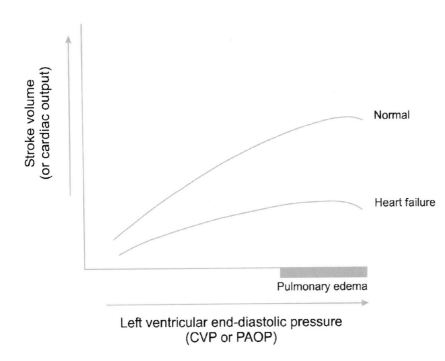

Stroke volume
(or cardiac output)

Normal

Heart failure

Pulmonary edema

Left ventricular end-diastolic pressure
(CVP or PAOP)

Fig. 9.2 The Starling curve. Demonstrating the Frank–Starling law of the heart: the heart ejects what it receives. Thus stroke volume increases with filling pressure. In heart failure the relationship shifts downward – increased ventricular filling fails to increase stroke volume and the high filling pressure eventually causes pulmonary edema. CVP: central venous pressure, PAOP: pulmonary artery occlusion pressure.

curve, we see that, if a patient becomes hypotensive but has an abnormally *high* CVP, something must be wrong with the ejection of the blood – either ischemia or perhaps diastolic dysfunction from some other cause.

Starling's law is in evidence when anesthetics cause venodilation, either directly or through inhibition of the sympathetic nervous system (there are some α_1 receptors on the venous side). This increased *venous capacity* causes peripheral pooling of blood away from the heart and reduces the venous pressure that ordinarily pushes blood back toward the right side of the heart. Functionally, this results in a reduced preload, limiting the stroke volume via Starling's law of the heart. Thus, managing anesthesia-induced hypotension with intravenous fluids makes a lot of sense. The fact this fluid must then be mobilized once the anesthetic effects are removed is another issue.

Remember that Starling's law is "length-dependent shortening" of heart muscle fibers and should not be confused with the energy-consuming *contractility* (although it is often difficult to distinguish these). For a given filling pressure, increasing contractility will shift the Starling curve upward, resulting in increased stroke volume (decreased end systolic volume). Such a shift can be achieved via β_1 receptors, either endogenously through the sympathetic nervous system and/or the baroreflex, or pharmacologically with many agents. Some anesthetic agents (particularly the volatile anesthetics) are direct myocardial depressants and will cause a dose-dependent downward shift and flattening of the Starling curve. Thus

Fig. 9.3 Starling's forces. Hydrostatic pressure is exerted by fluid, while proteins that cannot cross the vessel wall generate oncotic pressure. These forces exist on both sides of the vessel wall, but under physiologic conditions the intracapillary forces dominate over those exerted by the interstitium.

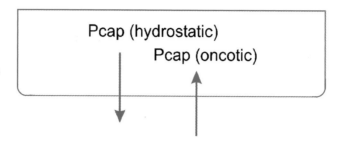

Pcap (hydrostatic)

Pcap (oncotic)

not only is there less central blood volume due to venodilation, more is required to achieve the same stroke volume.

Note in the blood pressure determinant diagram (Fig. 9.1), the parentheses surrounding the second "*Afterload*" under ejection fraction. Its effect here is actually the inverse. While increasing afterload directly raises blood pressure, increasing afterload reduces stroke volume by closing the aortic valve earlier in the ejection process. This partially explains why afterload reduction, e.g., via angiotensin converting enzyme (ACE) inhibitors benefits the patient in cardiac failure.

Other basic physical concepts to understand when thinking about the cardiovascular system include the following.

- *Compliance* The change in pressure resulting from a change in volume ($\Delta V/\Delta P$). As blood flows into a vessel, the highly compliant veins will greatly dilate to accommodate the volume, while the less compliant arteries dilate less, with a great increase in pressure. In many ways, compliance and resistance are simply the inverse of each other.
- *Starling's Forces* Not to be confused with his law of the heart (Dr. Starling, 1866–1927, was a busy man!). No vessel wall is entirely impermeable. Two main forces push and pull fluids across membranes (see Fig. 9.3). On the arterial side, the hydrostatic pressure on the luminal side of a capillary pushes fluid through the wall, while on the venous side, oncotic pressure of the proteins pulls fluids back into the vessel. You can readily imagine how increased capillary pressure and decreased oncotic pressure (low albumin) lead to the accumulation of fluids outside the capillary, i.e., edema.

So, putting it all together, the right atrium/ventricle receives oxygen-poor blood from the periphery and pumps it through the low resistance vascular bed of the lungs for a swap of carbon dioxide for oxygen. Meanwhile, the left atrium and ventricle stand by to receive the oxygenated blood and pump it on its way to the periphery. Upon taking leave of the heart, the blood travels through the aorta and peripheral arteries. The speed with which it is propelled forward depends not only on the cardiac output but also on the character of the arterial vessels. If hard and inelastic (an old aorta can have poor compliance; atheromatous vessels in the periphery offer high resistance), the stroke volume from a cardiac contraction will cause a substantial increase in pressure.

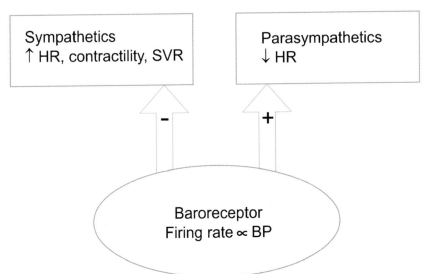

Fig. 9.4 Baroreflex. The baroreceptor in the carotid body fires in proportion to the blood pressure (more rapid with hypertension, slower with hypotension). Knowing the expected response (tachycardia with hypotension and vice versa), we recognize the baroreceptor must inhibit the sympathetics (less inhibition during hypotension) and stimulate the parasympathetics (less bradycardia with hypotension).

The venous side represents a quintessential low resistance bed. It accommodates large volumes of fluid with little rise in pressure, at least up to a point. A number of factors can increase the pressure and decrease flow in the vena cava: the surgeon with a hand in the abdomen, the uterus with a baby inside, the ventilator running up a high peak inspiratory and, consequently, intrathoracic pressure, the patient performing a Valsalva maneuver, the abdomen insufflated with gas for a laparoscopy, or the heart if it is stiff from diastolic dysfunction, or if it cannot expand because of fluid in the pericardial sac (tamponade).

Finally, we must briefly discuss the control mechanisms that keep everything running smoothly.

Blood pressure control

So blood pressure can take a major hit with decreases in preload (blood/fluid loss, venodilation), contractility and afterload. The body, however, has reflexes to try to fix this. For short-term blood pressure control, the baroreflex bears the brunt of the responsibility.

Baroreceptor

Located in the carotid sinus, the baroreceptor provides the most important immediate feedback mechanism for short-term control of blood pressure. These pressure receptors have a basal firing rate, stimulating the vagal center and inhibiting the vasomotor center (Fig. 9.4).

Hypertension increases the firing rate, amplifying the vagal effects. Conversely, hypotension results in *decreased* baroreceptor firing (a little counter-intuitive), resulting in reduced stimulation of the vagal centers and less inhibition (as opposed to stimulation) of the vasomotor center. The end-result is increased sympathetic outflow, resulting in increased heart rate, contractility, and SVR with decreased venous capacity. This reflex requires an intact sympathetic nervous system, that is, one that has not been destroyed by the ravages of diabetes, blocked with neuraxial anesthesia, or depleted with illicit drugs, e.g., cocaine.

Atrial stretch receptors

Stretch on the atria, particularly the sinoatrial node, results in reflex vasodilation and decreased blood pressure, as well as increased heart rate. Simultaneously, atrial stretch receptors elicit the *Bainbridge reflex*[3] with a vagal afferent to the medulla and efferents through the vagus and sympathetics to increase heart rate and contractility.

Chemoreceptor

Located in the carotid and aortic bodies, the chemoreceptors are stimulated by decreasing oxygen and increasing carbon dioxide and hydrogen ion. They affect the vasomotor center to increase blood pressure, as well as stimulate breathing. Of less importance, receptors in the ventricles elicit a vasodepressor (vasodilation and bradycardia) response to decreased ventricular volume (vasovagal reflex) or certain chemical or mechanical stimuli (Bezold–Jarisch reflex).[4]

Long-term control

Long-term blood pressure control occurs through the kidney and aldosterone, renin, and angiotensin, which alter the volume of fluid in the system and can adjust vascular resistances as well.

Anesthesia in the patient with cardiovascular disease

Hypertension

When we do not know the etiology, we hide behind the technical term "essential." Thus, we call "essential" the hypertension afflicting some 95% of patients. The pathophysiology of essential hypertension is probably multi-factorial including renal, vascular, cardiac, and neurohumoral factors – and reflex control problems thrown in for good measure.

Chronic hypertension leads to left ventricular hypertrophy with consequent stiffening of the ventricle. A "stiffer," less compliant ventricle will exhibit a large rise in intraventricular pressure during diastole. This increased diastolic pressure (wall tension) both increases myocardial oxygen demand and limits coronary

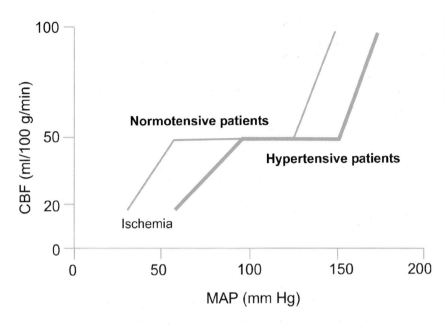

Fig. 9.5 Cerebral autoregulation curve. Cerebral blood flow (CBF) is maintained over a range of mean arterial pressures (MAP). The curve shifts with chronic hypertension, increasing the potential for inadequate cerebral blood flow with marginal MAP. Ischemia results when the CBF falls below 20 mL/100 g/min.

perfusion. All organ perfusion depends on the upstream and downstream pressures. Thus, for the coronary perfusion pressure (CorPP):

CorPP = DBP − RAP or LVEDP

where DBP = diastolic blood pressure (because the majority of coronary perfusion occurs during diastole), RAP = right atrial pressure (where the coronaries empty, measured as central venous pressure, CVP), and LVEDP = left ventricular end-diastolic pressure. With a stiff left ventricle, LVEDP may exceed RAP and limit coronary perfusion, particularly in the subendocardium. This combination leads to an increased risk of myocardial ischemia (oxygen supply < demand). In addition to its deleterious effects on the heart, chronic hypertension leads to aortic, cerebral, and peripheral vascular disease, as well as strokes and renal dysfunction.

In all patients, particularly those we are going to anesthetize, we worry about cerebral perfusion. The cerebral vasculature autoregulates to maintain a stable blood flow over a range of mean arterial pressures. Chronic hypertension causes a rightward shift of this cerebral autoregulation curve (see Fig. 9.5). An unfortunate side effect of this shift is intolerance of low blood pressure. That is, a normotensive patient can maintain cerebral blood flow down to a MAP of 50 mmHg; with chronic hypertension, such a MAP might result in decreased cerebral perfusion and possibly ischemia (decreased CNS function or even a stroke). While a conscious patient might complain of dizziness and perhaps become confused, under general anesthesia we find it difficult to assess the adequacy of cerebral perfusion.

Thus, we apply a general, albeit conservative, rule of thumb: maintain a patient's blood pressure within 20% of their baseline pressure.

The anesthetic management of hypertension includes the following:

(i) Pre-operative control of blood pressure. We have data showing that grossly hypertensive patients do poorly peri-operatively; we have no data that would enable us to pinpoint the optimum of controlled hypertension.

(ii) Continuation of anti-hypertensive medication in the peri-operative period, with the possible exception of ACE inhibitors, which have been linked to refractory hypotension intra-operatively.

(iii) Intra-operative control of blood pressure swings. Hypertensive patients are often volume depleted from chronic vasoconstriction or because they take diuretics. Most anesthetics are vasodilators, and blood pressure can fall precipitously. Furthermore, the presence of anti-hypertensive drugs and some anesthetics may interfere with the normal reflex response to hypotension. As already mentioned, hypotension presents a particular risk to hypertensive patients because they require increased diastolic pressure to maintain coronary perfusion and may have impaired cerebral autoregulation.

Ischemic heart disease

Patients with ischemic heart disease face significant risks when undergoing anesthesia and surgical procedures. In our pre-operative assessment, we must weigh measures to protect them from peri-operative ischemia (see Pre-operative evaluation). Diagnosing ischemia by electrocardiography (ST-segment depression) can be difficult if a bundle branch block pattern obscures ST-segment changes. Transesophageal echocardiography (TEE), which is minimally invasive (but unpleasant if awake), can be quite helpful as it reveals wall motion abnormalities, an early sign of ventricular dysfunction from coronary insufficiency. TEE requires a skilled observer and expensive equipment (see Monitoring).

If we suspect ischemia, remember physiology: ischemia means oxygen supply does not meet demand. By looking at the factors affecting supply and demand, we can try to improve conditions (Table 9.1).

First, consider *supply*. Because the coronary arteries are perfused during diastole, we want to maximize diastolic time (lower heart rate) and coronary perfusion pressure (see above). For each amount of blood that gets through, we want it to contain as much oxygen as possible (see oxygen content equation in Anesthesia and the lung). Surprisingly, the optimal hematocrit is actually only 30 mg/dL; at higher concentrations, fluidity of blood decreases.

Now for *demand*. Cardiac contraction is "expensive" in an oxygen consumption sense, and the more contractions, the more "expense." Thus, tachycardia has a dramatic impact on the supply : demand ratio, increasing oxygen consumption while at the same time reducing its supply. For this reason, heart rate reduction is a

Table 9.1. Factors affecting myocardial oxygen supply and demand

Factors increasing supply

↓ Heart rate

↑ Diastolic blood pressure

↓ Intraventricular pressure

↑ Oxygen saturation

↑ [Hemoglobin]

Factors decreasing demand

↓ Heart rate

↓ Wall tension

↓ Contractility

primary target during ischemic episodes. In addition, myocardial oxygen demand increases with increasing wall tension and, more importantly, contractility.

As of this writing, peri-operative beta-receptor blockade receives much attention. It may have the potential to reduce cardiac deaths and complications (see Pharmacology).

Pacemaker/AICD

More and more patients are presenting with these life-saving devices (ACID, automatic internal cardiac defibrillator) in place for heart rhythm disturbances (see Pre-operative evaluation: Pacemaker/AICD for advance evaluation). Intra-operatively, there are general rules for surgery in these patients:

(i) Enlist the help of cardiology colleagues to check on the pacer function following the operation.

(ii) Have a magnet on hand. This nifty low-tech device reverts most pacemakers into a back-up paced-only mode at a rate dependent on the manufacturer, program, and remaining battery life.

(iii) Avoid electromagnetic interference. We do not want the pacemaker to become part of the electrocautery circuit, so we consider the route between the surgical site and the electrocautery grounding pad and make sure it does not cross the pacemaker or its leads.

(iv) With rate-responsive pacemakers, we might avoid agents that fool the device into thinking its owner is running a marathon (succinylcholine-induced fasciculations, shivering).

(v) Disable AICDs to prevent inappropriate shock when the device is confused by electrocautery.

(vi) Keep electrolytes normal, particularly K^+ and Mg^{2+}.

Following conclusion of the operation, the pacer may require reprogramming, and the AICD should be reactivated.

Congestive heart failure

Congestive heart failure (CHF) describes a heart that is not pumping well. Ordinarily, the heart dilates to accept blood at a low filling pressure, then propels it forward forcefully with each contraction. CHF can result from pathology at several points in the pump's function:

(i) Poor *ventricular compliance* A non-compliant ventricle, as may occur with ischemia or hypertrophy, will exhibit substantial increases in pressure at even "normal" filling volumes. This will impede ventricular filling and increase the pressure in the venous system. In approximately one-third of CHF patients, this *diastolic dysfunction* predominates as the mechanism for their disease.

(ii) The descending limb of *Starling's curve* Though a bit controversial, there may be a point at which further increasing diastolic filling actually results in a *decreasing* stroke volume. Here, substantial increases in ventricular pressure can result in pulmonary congestion and edema. A reduction in preload can move the heart back to the more functional side of the curve (see Fig. 9.2) and reduce the filling pressure sufficient to alleviate pulmonary congestion.

(iii) *Contractility* In Fig. 9.2, the Starling curve of the CHF patient resides lower and runs flatter than normal, reflecting the high filling pressures required to generate even a marginal stroke volume.

(iv) *Afterload* Increased afterload is the most common cause of hypertension. The increased force of contraction required to eject against this afterload is deleterious to a failing heart.

The importance of these influences suggests the current treatment regimen for the most common cause of CHF, left ventricular systolic dysfunction, namely inotropic support with digoxin, diuretics to decrease preload, and afterload reduction with an ACE inhibitor.

Cardiovascular problems during anesthesia

Hypotension

Picture the acutely hypotensive, tachycardic patient (BP 80/50 HR 120 bpm), a fairly common observation. How should you go about treating this patient? After the ABCs,[5] we recommend a physiologic approach, rather than a mnemonic laundry list of possible causes. First, there are three main ways a patient can become hypotensive: low preload (not enough blood to push forward through the system), low contractility (inadequate force pushing the blood), and low resistance (dilated vascular bed). Other categories are less common and include severe bradycardia, lack of atrial kick, and valvular anomalies, to name a few. To distinguish between these, we start with situational awareness. Did the cross-clamp just come off the

Table 9.2. Differentiating causes of hypotension

	CVP	CO	SVR	Treatment
Low preload: hemorrhage, increased intra-abdominal pressure, sympathetic block, anesthetics	↓	↓ ↔	↑	Fluids; Trendelenburg's position
Low contractility: ischemia, CHF, anesthetics	↑	↓	↑ ↔	Inotrope; ? vasodilator/diuretic; oxygen
Low SVR: anaphylaxis, sepsis, spinal shock, anesthetics	↓	↑	↓	Vasoconstriction, e.g., α_1 agonist

Notes: Until the preload is very low, there is usually sufficient cardiac reserve (increased heart rate and contractility) to maintain cardiac output. With low contractility, initial baroreflex-mediated stimulation will cause vasoconstriction – not such a good idea in a heart already having difficulty ejecting! Over time, this response dissipates, and SVR returns toward normal. CO = cardiac output.

aorta? Did we just induce a sympathectomy with a high spinal anesthetic? Add to that a quick physical examination to rule out abnormal rhythm or valvular or cardiac dysfunction and review of the patient's medical history (chronic CHF or recent myocardial infarction (MI)?. If these do not lead to a high-probability diagnosis, invasive monitoring may be indicated.

The invasive monitors we have available, in addition to the arterial catheter for blood pressure monitoring, include:
- filling pressure as an inference of ventricular volume/preload: central venous pressure (CVP), pulmonary capillary wedge pressure (PCWP);
- cardiac output: thermodilution via a pulmonary artery catheter (PAC).

For example, consider the hypotensive, tachycardic patient above. Assume a CVP of 1 mmHg (normal 5–12 mmHg) and cardiac output of 6.5 L/min. A low filling pressure (low preload) translates into low ventricular volume – but contractility appears to be good (a cardiac output of 6.5 L/min is not consistent with a poorly contracting heart). With a look at the systemic vascular resistance (SVR) equation above, we see that a low MAP (small numerator) and high cardiac output (denominator) implies a very low SVR. The baroreflex, though, should be railing against the low BP and *raising* the SVR – we cannot measure the baroreflex activity but assume that it is straining to raise resistance, without success. Thus, our attention is drawn to vasodilation (via endotoxin as in septic shock, or blockade of sympathetic outflow as in spinal shock or neuraxial anesthesia).

Such a physiologic approach allows tailoring of intervention to the specific problem. While intravenous fluid administration is routinely our first choice in a hypotensive patient – particularly in the post-operative setting – and proves the correct choice 99 times out of 100, it does no favor for the patient hypotensive from CHF. Thus, with an unclear etiology or a troubling response to initial treatment, invasive monitoring may be helpful (Table 9.2).

Table 9.3. Causes of intra-operative hypertension

Underlying hypertension (exacerbated by missing anti-hypertensive doses while awaiting surgery)
- rebound hypertension (especially from missing beta blockers or clonidine)
- pre-eclampsia

Elevated catecholamines
- anxiety
- inadequate anesthetic depth for level of stimulation (surgery, laryngoscopy, emergence)
- iatrogenic (drug error, inadvertent intravascular injection or absorption)
- drugs (cocaine, monoamine oxidase inhibitors (MAOIs), ephedra)
- bladder distension
- pheochromocytoma

Reflexes
- hypoxia
- hypercarbia
- Cushing's reflex (from elevated ICP)
- autonomic hyperreflexia (from spinal reflexes after cord transection)

Elevated preload (volume overload)

Elevated afterload
- drugs (decongestants)
- aortic cross-clamp

Rare events
- malignant hyperthermia
- thyroid storm
- delirium tremens

We see from the table that the typical general inhalation anesthetic can affect blood pressure from top to bottom, decreasing preload by venous pooling, decreasing contractility by a direct negative inotropic effect on the heart, decreasing SVR by depressing sympathetic outflow and, with some agents, even decreasing the baroreceptor reflex. The treatment of hypotension under anesthesia – when not attributed to primary heart disease, hypovolemia from hemorrhage or sepsis – still consists of "filling up the tank" by giving fluids, lightening anesthesia to improve cardiac function. and giving sympthomimetic drugs, such as ephedrine, to raise SVR and contractility.

Arrhythmias

Rhythm disturbances occur in up to 70% of patients subjected to general anesthesia. Fortunately, the majority of these, in the otherwise healthy patient, are benign and transient. A number of factors can be blamed: the effects of anesthetic agents on the SA and AV nodes, peri-operative ischemia, and increased sympathetic activity during light anesthesia, e.g., laryngoscopy, hypoxemia, and hypercarbia (not uncommon during induction of general anesthesia). In addition to adhering to ACLS protocols, potential triggers must be sought and eliminated: correct ventilation, alter anesthetic agent selection (no halothane), increase oxygenation, deepen anesthetic, etc.

Hypertension

The differential diagnosis of intraoperative hypertension is lengthy, but should be approached by considering the patient and procedure first (Table 9.3).

Management of intra-operative hypertension should focus on three things:

(i) Fix the underlying problem: correct anesthetic depth, treat hypercarbia, drain the bladder, etc.

(ii) Where correction is not possible: treat according to the physiologic derangement. For example, volume overload should not be treated with beta-blockade nor anxiety with diuretics.

(iii) Consider the time course of the treatment: if a patient's hypertension results from a transient surgical stimulus, a long-acting anti-hypertensive may cause refractory hypotension when the stimulus ends.

See the pharmacology section to review a selection of the myriad anti-hypertensive agents at our disposal.

NOTES

1. You might (at least the engineers in the crowd) recognize this equation as a corollary to Ohm's Law ($V = IR$) with blood pressure drop over the body circuit replacing the voltage drop, cardiac output replacing current (I), and SVR in the role of resistance (R). The "$\times 80$" part corrects the units into the dubious "dynes s cm^{-5}".

2. Actually more correctly the (Otto) Frank – (Hermann) Straub – (Ernest) Starling law of the heart – to give credit where credit is due.

3. Francis Arthur Bainbridge (1874–1921), an English physiologist particularly interested in the physiology of exercise.

4. Albert von Bezold (1836–1868) described the slowing of the heart in response to veratrine (an irritant). Upon his untimely death at age 32 from rheumatic heart disease, his work was greatly furthered by Austrian Adolph Jarisch, Jr. (1891–1965).

5. Airway, Breathing, Circulation.

10

Anesthesia and the lung

> And the Lord God formed man from the dust of the ground and breathed into his nostrils the breath of life; and man became a living soul
>
> (Genesis 2;7)

The concept of breath and soul reverberates through many languages in which spirit and breath share overlapping meanings. For example, in English, to *inspire* can have a physiological or psychological connotation, while to *expire* can mean nothing more than to exhale, or it can describe the moment when your spirit leaves you with your last breath. In anesthesia, we deal with both; on the one hand, the breath that needs to be provided for patients who cannot breathe by themselves and, on the other hand, the spirit – in a larger sense – which we subdue with drugs. Small wonder, then, that the linkage of breath and life gives us awesome responsibilities. In our practice no function is more important than ventilation, and no organ more integral to our practice than the lungs. Failure of ventilation has always been, and continues to be, the single most important cause of anesthesia-related mortality. An understanding of basic pulmonary physiology and pathophysiology therefore, is vital to the safe practice of anesthesia.

Basic pulmonary physiology

Purpose of breathing

Breathing brings in oxygen necessary for cellular respiration and eliminates the resulting carbon dioxide. If oxygen supply does not meet demand, desperate cells revert to anaerobic metabolism, resulting in lactic acidosis.[1] Our oxygen requirement depends on the metabolic rate, but for a resting individual 3 mL O_2/kg/min, should suffice. Meanwhile, we generate CO_2 at a rate dependent on the respiratory quotient "R:"

$$R = \frac{\dot{V}_{CO_2}}{\dot{V}_{O_2}}$$

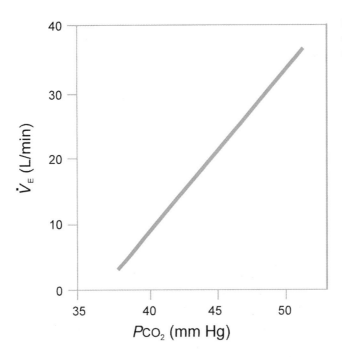

Fig. 10.1 Ventilatory response to changing $PaCO_2$. $\dot{V}_E$ = exhaled minute ventilation.

where $\dot{V}_{CO_2}$ and $\dot{V}_{O_2}$ are the minute production of carbon dioxide and consumption of oxygen, respectively. R depends on the energy source (carbohydrates, proteins, fat). R approaches 1 in several conditions including pregnancy and patients on total peripheral nutrition (TPN), but we usually peg it at 0.8.

Control of breathing

Can you commit suicide by simply not breathing or by willing your heart to stop? Even though we have voluntary muscular control over ventilation, we cannot stop breathing. We are hard-wired so that, in response to rising carbon dioxide tensions in the medulla, carbon dioxide-sensitive neurons stimulate ventilation to keep the arterial partial pressure of CO_2 ($PaCO_2$) near 40 mmHg. In physiological sleep, they let the $PaCO_2$ drift up to 45 mmHg, while in pregnancy, they are reset by the controller to maintain 30 mmHg. Within physiological limits, ventilation and $PaCO_2$ (Fig. 10.1) keep a linear relationship.

We can restrain the center pharmacologically with opioids or deep inhalation anesthesia. In some diseases resulting in high $PaCO_2$, the respiratory center fatigues permanently, and these "CO_2 retainers" must then rely on hypoxemia to drive their ventilation.

Perhaps surprisingly, oxygenation is not detected in the brain at all, but rather is sensed by peripheral chemoreceptors in the carotid and aortic bodies. These receptors do not really kick in until the PaO_2 falls below about 60 mmHg. Thus, our "CO_2-retaining" patients with chronic obstructive pulmonary disease (COPD) are not only chronically hypercarbic, they are also (at least borderline) hypoxemic. We often hear it said that such a patient will become apneic if given supplemental oxygen. Please do not take this to mean that, in an emergency, oxygen should be withheld from a hypoxemic patient for fear of apnea! Instead, give oxygen and ventilate the patient's lungs. Once on top of the emergency, turn down the FiO_2 step by step and remind the patient to breathe (no small task) until the oxygen saturation falls to a point where hypoxic drive takes effect. Similarly, when weaning these patients from mechanical ventilation, they might not start to breathe until returned to the hypoxic and hypercarbic state to which they are accustomed (another curse of smoking).

Mechanics of ventilation

Spontaneous ventilation at rest involves generating negative intrathoracic pressure (by lowering the diaphragm and expanding the chest wall), causing air to be drawn into the lungs. This requires that the upper airway remains patent. In the presence of an obstruction, e.g., tongue, mass, mechanical, we observe retractions, particularly around the clavicles and the jugular notch and, in children, the intercostal spaces. An early sign is a *tracheal tug*, a little downward movement of the larynx with each inspiration. A reliable sign of airway obstruction, the tracheal tug signals the recruitment of accessory muscles to maintain gas exchange. Similarly, pulmonary cripples (advanced emphysema) and patients still partially paralyzed after anesthesia will show a tracheal tug. Hypoxemic patients weakened by drugs or muscle disease require immediate assisted ventilation with bag and mask and, if necessary, establishment of a patent airway.

At rest, exhalation should be passive and, if it is not, consider asthma or airway obstruction.

The work of breathing

The medullary centers control the $PaCO_2$ by altering the minute ventilation ($\dot{V}_E$):

$$\dot{V}_E = V_T \times f$$

where V_T = tidal volume and f = respiratory rate. How these parameters change to maintain minute ventilation depends on the work of breathing. Because inhaling requires the work of muscles, it is "costly," in an energy expenditure sense, to breathe. In general, a few large breaths are more efficient than many small ones because all breaths must move the same amount of deadspace volume (about 150 mL for the average adult, see below). Endotracheal tubes offer much resistance and can greatly increase the work of breathing. The ventilator will ease this burden by doing the inspiratory work for the patient. Just as with all other muscles, disuse leads to reduced strength and stamina. Several investigators continue to study the optimal amount of respiratory muscle loading to prevent muscle atrophy and weaning difficulties.

Patients with low pulmonary *compliance*, e.g., pulmonary fibrosis, tend to breathe rapidly with low tidal volumes because of the great work required to expand a stiff lung. Compliance (C) describes the relationship between volume (V) and pressure (P) in any enclosed space (lung, cardiac ventricle):

$$C = \frac{\Delta V}{\Delta P}$$

Conversely, a patient with high *airway resistance* cannot move air rapidly through the bronchial tree and tends to breathe slowly, which decreases turbulence. The resulting shift toward laminar movement of air increases flow.

Since resistance decreases as the fourth power of the radius, we can easily see why even a small amount of bronchospasm so drastically affects air movement, and why babies with subglottic edema present us with such great difficulties.

Matching of ventilation and perfusion

All the tubing leading to the alveoli – trachea, large bronchi, endotracheal tube – serves only as a conduit. These make up the deadspace volume: areas with bi-directional airflow but no gas exchange. There are three types of deadspace:
- physiologic – areas of the normal lung with ventilation but no perfusion – as found in the apices;
- anatomic – trachea and bronchi, which lack alveoli altogether;
- apparatus – the endotracheal tube and other pieces of tubing with bidirectional gas flow.

An endotracheal tube will decrease the anatomic dead space generated by the pharynx, nose, and mouth. Applying a face mask will increase deadspace, but an anesthesia breathing circuit will add relatively little to the deadspace as long as the valves in the circuit function normally. The deadspace to tidal volume ratio is measured as:

$$V_D/V_T = (P_ACO_2 - P_{\bar{E}}CO_2)/P_ACO_2$$

where V_D = deadspace volume, P_ACO_2 = alveolar CO_2 and $P_{\bar{E}}CO_2$ = mixed expired CO_2. A normal V_D/V_T ratio should not exceed 0.3.

When pulmonary arterial blood manages to pass through the lungs without picking up oxygen or delivering carbon dioxide, we are referring to shunting. A shunt wastes perfusion. Typically, the difference between arterial and end-expired gases increases when ventilation and perfusion are mismatched, either owing to deadspace ventilation (inspired gas returns without having picked up carbon dioxide or delivered oxygen) or to shunting (pulmonary arterial blood bypasses alveoli and then dumps blood high in CO_2 and low in O_2 into the pulmonary venous blood, see Fig. 10.2). Even normal lungs have some deadspace ventilation

Fig. 10.2 Ventilation–perfusion mismatch. The ideal is perfect matching of ventilation and perfusion ($V/Q=1$). To the far left, the numerator falls to zero ($V=0$), representing no ventilation but plenty of perfusion; this is termed shunt. Deadspace ventilation is the opposite. Thus deadspace ventilation and shunt represent the extremes on the continuum of V/Q matching. See text.

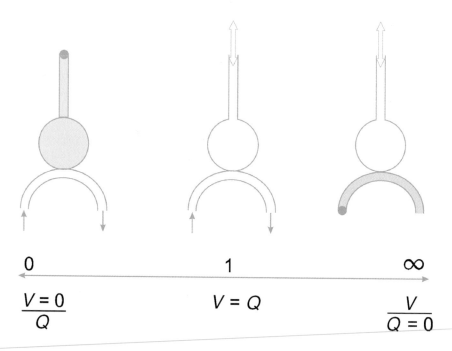

and shunting. When either becomes excessive, we refer to a V/Q mismatch evident in abnormal blood gas values.

Tissue oxygenation

Once we get both air and blood into the lungs, oxygen must traverse the alveolar membrane. Oxygen diffusion across this membrane depends on the Fick[2] Equation:

$$Diffusion = \frac{SA}{T} \times D \times (P_{alv} - P_{bld})$$

where SA = surface area of the alveoli (decreased in emphysema); T = membrane thickness (increased with pulmonary edema), D = diffusion constant for a given gas,[3] and $P_{alv} - P_{bld}$ = the gas pressure difference across the membrane dividing alveolus from blood.

After traversing the alveolar and capillary wall membrane, oxygen dissolves in plasma (not much; $0.003 \times PaO_2$) and binds with hemoglobin (a bunch), and the arterial oxygen content (CaO_2) becomes

$$CaO_2 = 1.34 \times [Hgb] \times SaO_2 + 0.003 \times PaO_2$$

where CaO_2 = volume of oxygen in 100 mL blood, Hgb = hemoglobin concentration, and SaO_2 = arterial hemoglobin saturation with oxygen.

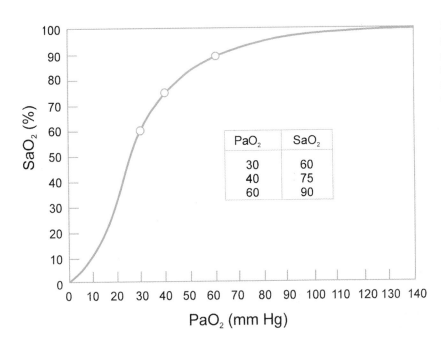

PaO$_2$	SaO$_2$
30	60
40	75
60	90

Fig. 10.3 The oxyhemoglobin dissociation curve for normal adult hemoglobin. SaO$_2$ is saturation of hemoglobin with oxygen; PaO$_2$ is partial pressure of oxygen in arterial blood.

Oxyhemoglobin dissociation curve

The amount of oxygen bound to hemoglobin depends on the qualities of the hemoglobin molecule. The familiar oxyhemoglobin dissociation curve appears in Fig. 10.3. Observe the steep part of the curve where small changes in PaO$_2$ result in large shifts in saturation. The point of 50% saturation (P$_{50}$) provides a helpful reference. In adults, it hovers around 26 mmHg (the hemoglobin will be 50% saturated with oxygen at a PaO$_2$ of 26 mmHg). The left shift of fetal hemoglobin brings its P$_{50}$ to 19 mmHg.

A simple mnemonic helps to define several points on the oxyhemoglobin dissociation curve: 30–60; 60–90; 40–75 (Fig. 10.3). It does not sound much like a mnemonic, but put it to a beat and it works quite well. The first number of each pair cites the PaO$_2$, followed by the SaO$_2$. We use this to estimate (roughly) the PaO$_2$ from the SpO$_2$ (obtained from the pulse oximeter). A PaO$_2$ of 60 mmHg or less defines hypoxemia (SpO$_2$ ~90%), and 40 mmHg is the normal mixed venous PO$_2$.

Four factors influence the position of the oxyhemoglobin dissociation curve. For ease of memorization, we cite those factors that shift the curve to the right: *increasing* temperature, CO$_2$, H$^+$, and 2,3-diphosphoglycerate (DPG). Remember pH decreases with increasing [H$^+$].

Alveolar air equation

The PO$_2$ we expect to find in arterial blood depends, in large part, on the inspired concentration. Oxygen makes up approximately 21% of the volume of dry air. If we assume the ambient (sea level) pressure to be 760 mmHg, the partial pressure of oxygen in dry air would be 160 mmHg (760×0.21). The warm and moist airways add water (water vapor pressure is temperature-dependent, and at 37 °C it is 47 mmHg). Thus, breathing room air, our inspired oxygen concentration (PiO_2) on its way through the nose and upper airway will be diluted by water vapor:

$$PiO_2 = (760 - 47) \times 0.21 = 150 \, mmHg$$

Once it arrives in the alveolus, this inspired oxygen will be diluted by carbon dioxide and taken up into the bloodstream. Summarized mathematically,[4] the resulting equation is too cumbersome for clinical application. Instead, we use the approximation commonly referred to as the alveolar air equation:

$$P_A O_2 = P_i O_2 - \frac{P_A C O_2}{R}$$

where the "A" subscript denotes alveolar gas.

If we take the trouble of calculating for a person breathing room air ($PiO_2 = 150$ mmHg), assuming $R = 0.8$ and $P_A CO_2 = 40$ mmHg, we arrive at a $P_A O_2$ of about 100 mmHg. You can easily see that many factors can change the results: altitude, retention or rebreathing of CO_2, changing the concentration of oxygen in the inspired gas, changing the respiratory quotient, or changing the patient's temperature.

Clinical relevance of the oxyhemoglobin dissociation curve

Notice on the curve (Fig. 10.3), if a patient has an oxyhemoglobin saturation of 100%, we know that the PaO_2 must be at least 100 mmHg, but it could be anywhere from about 100 to 600 mmHg or more! We see the importance when administering supplemental oxygen in two different scenarios that follow.

The hypoxemic patient

When a patient becomes hypoxemic, we first apply supplemental oxygen. Wonderfully, the patient's saturation usually responds. Should it fall again, we can simply increase the inspired oxygen concentration once again – but we are not solving the problem. The adequate saturation may lull us into an inappropriate sense of security regarding the well-being of the patient.

Assume this patient requires 50% inspired oxygen to maintain a SpO_2 of 90%, much less than we would expect with that FiO_2. We estimate the degree of the oxygenation problem by looking at the difference between the alveolar and arterial oxygen concentrations. With a SpO_2 of 90%, we can assume the PaO_2 to be around 60 mmHg (from Fig. 10.3).

Next, we need to know what the alveolar concentration of oxygen would be in the patient breathing 50% oxygen. The alveolar air equation comes to our aid. We estimate $P_A CO_2$ and R to be 40 mmHg and 0.8, respectively.

$$P_A O_2 = F_i O_2 \times (P_B - P_{H_2 O}) - \frac{P_A CO_2}{R}$$

$$P_A O_2 = 0.50 \times (760 - 47) - \frac{40}{0.8} = 306\, mmHg$$

Therefore, we would expect the PaO_2 to be close to 300 mmHg instead of the observed 60 mmHg. This "A-a difference" (often mislabeled an A – a gradient) may be due to a problem with oxygen diffusion and/or matching of ventilation and perfusion (V/Q). In healthy patients some 4% of the venous blood will manage to make it through a right (venous blood in the pulmonary artery) to left (arterial blood in the pulmonary vein) shunt. Thus, normally we expect to see a slightly lower partial pressure of oxygen in arterial blood than in alveolar gas. However, a patient requiring 50% inspired oxygen to barely maintain a SpO_2 of 90% should worry us greatly.

If a patient is hypoxemic on room air, giving supplemental oxygen is a great first step, but the *source* of the hypoxemia should be sought and appropriately treated.

Conscious sedation

The patient receiving intravenous sedation presents another situation in which the alveolar air equation can help. Some physicians routinely place these patients on supplemental oxygen by nasal cannula, resulting in a PaO_2 of 150 mmHg or more (well into the flat part of the oxyhemoglobin dissociation curve: Fig. 10.3). If the patient now hypoventilates, his $PaCO_2$ will rise and PaO_2 will fall, but his SpO_2 can stay deceptively normal. Thus, *not* giving supplemental oxygen (to a patient with normal oxygenation) will make the SpO_2 a sensitive indicator of respiratory depression. Once a drop in saturation occurs, we need to treat the patient's hypoventilation.

Studies of pulmonary function

Spirometry

Pulmonary function tests (PFTs) are rarely indicated in preparation for anesthesia, though they can tell us whether a patient with severe lung disease has been optimally prepared. Pulmonary restrictive and obstructive diseases worry us. Short of treating infection, we cannot do much about restrictive disease; however, it can co-exist with obstructive bronchospasm, which is common and can be treated with bronchodilators. Of the many pulmonary function studies, we pay particular attention to forced vital capacity (FVC). FVC values below 15 mL/kg give rise to great concern. How much the patient can exhale in 1 second (FEV_1), and whether this can be improved by bronchodilators determines obstructive

Table 10.1. Pulmonary function test interpretation

	FEV_1	FVC	FEV_1/FVC
Normal	>80%	>80%	>0.8
Obstruction	↓	↔ ↓	↓
Restriction	↓	↓	↔ ↑

% of predicted; FEV_1 = forced expiratory volume in 1 s.
FVC = forced vital capacity.
In obstructive disease, FVC may decline due to air trapping.

disease. Typically, PFT results are reported as "% of predicted," based on population studies that consider the patient's height, age, and gender. We accept values of at least 80% predicted as normal. With obstructive disease, the patient experiences airway closure during exhalation, measured as a low FEV_1 (Table 10.1). With advanced disease and air trapping, the FVC might also decline, though not as much as the FEV_1, thus the hallmark of obstructive disease is a reduced ratio of FEV_1 to FVC. With age, this ratio declines as well (to perhaps 0.7), so again we look at the percentage predicted. Flow volume loops (Fig. 10.4) can also be helpful.

Arterial blood gas analysis

When we call for an analysis of arterial blood gases (ABG), we are really asking about the function of two organs: lungs and kidneys. An ABG reports the partial pressures of oxygen and carbon dioxide in arterial blood, both clearly related to lung function, but also provides the pH and bicarbonate concentration, which tells us something about how the kidneys are handling non-volatile acids and bases.

In the laboratory, the ABG values are corrected to 37 °C. This facilitates interpretation of data because of the complexities introduced by temperature changes: in addition to a direct effect on pH, both the dissociation constants and solubility of gases are temperature dependent. For example, a $PaCO_2$ of 40 mmHg at 37 °C, will drop to 25 mmHg when temperature falls 10 degrees. The total carbon dioxide content stays the same, but the distribution of the components of the CO_2–carbonic acid–bicarbonate complex has changed (see below). Thus, if not corrected in the laboratory, a drop in temperature from 37 °C to 27 °C would raise the reported pH of the blood sample from 7.4 to about 7.54.

Oxygen

The lab reports the partial pressure of oxygen in arterial blood as PaO_2 in mmHg, and the saturation of arterial hemoglobin with oxygen as % SaO_2. Most ABG analyzers *calculate* the SaO_2 based on a standard, adult oxyhemoglobin dissociation curve. When there is doubt regarding the actual saturation, e.g., in the patient

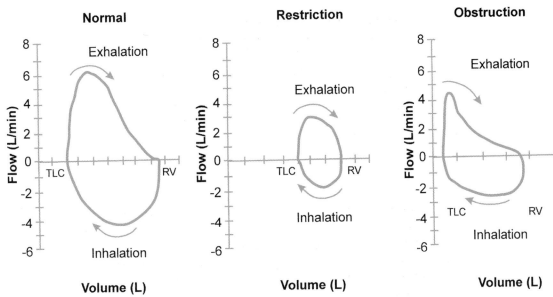

Normal

Restriction

Obstruction

Fig. 10.4 Flow volume loop obtained in a normal patient, compared with those with restrictive and obstructive pulmonary diseases. With restriction, the flow volume loop has a slightly more convex shape and small volume. Note the rapid decline in the flow rate in the patient with moderate obstruction. TLC = total lung capacity; RV = residual volume. To read these loops, we must keep in mind that the x-axis is conventionally written backwards, with the 0 for volume to the *right*, and that inhalation is the area below the x-axis, and exhalation above.

with suspected carbon monoxide inhalation, we must order co-oximetry, which analyzes the transmission of several wavelengths of light, the better to distinguish reduced from oxygenated hemoglobin, as well as met- and carboxyhemoglobins. Please observe the convention of writing SaO_2 for the laboratory calculation of arterial hemoglobin saturation, SpO_2 for the estimation of this value by pulse oximetry, and specify SaO_2 by co-oximetry if available. These values are rarely, if ever, identical but usually agree within a percent or so.

Carbon dioxide

Carbon dioxide in blood affects the pH because CO_2 in an aqueous medium (i.e. blood) will form carbonic acid, which dissociates into bicarbonate and hydrogen ions:

$$CO_2 + H_2O \leftrightarrow H_2CO_3 \leftrightarrow H^+ + HCO_3^-$$

We often describe this relationship with *Henderson Hasselbalch's*[5] equation:

$$pH = pKa + \log\left(\frac{HCO_3^-}{PCO_2 \times 0.03}\right)$$

where pKa = the dissociation constant for carbonic acid ($\sim$6.1), that is, the pH at which 50% of the weak carbonic acid is ionized into equal amounts of HCO_3^- and H_2CO_3 (for which $PCO_2 \times 0.03$ is substituted). Thus the *ratio* of bicarbonate to PCO_2 determines pH, not their individual concentrations.

From this equation, we see that if we add carbon dioxide, the pH drops (respiratory acidosis). The interaction of CO_2 with water will lead to the generation

Table 10.2. Bicarbonate response to acute or chronic respiratory disturbances

	The $^1 2^4 6$ Rule of Ten	
	Change in bicarbonate, during hypercapnea above 40 mmHg	Change in bicarbonate during hypocapnea below 40 mmHg
Acute respiratory disturbance	**Up 1** mmol/L for every **10** mmHg PaCO$_2$ ↑	**Down 2** mmol/L for every **10** mmHg PaCO$_2$ ↓
Chronic respiratory disturbance	**Up 4** mmol/L for every **10** mmHg PaCO$_2$ ↑	**Down 6** mmol/L for every **10** mmHg PaCO$_2$ ↓

of carbonic acid, which will lower the pH while increasing bicarbonate, without which the pH would be even lower. Slowly (over 1–2 days), the kidneys retain extra bicarbonate to further offset the acidosis, although never completely correcting it. When faced with an ABG demonstrating respiratory acidosis (decreased pH and increased PCO$_2$), we can use the 1–2–4–6 Rule of Ten (see Table 10.2), which simply says that the indicated acute or chronic respiratory disturbance will cause the bicarbonate to change. If that change did not take place or is exaggerated, we need to look for metabolic explanations.

Bicarbonate

The addition of acids, e.g., keto acids in diabetes, will also lower the pH. From Henderson Hasselbalch's equation, we predict that the addition of hydrogen ions (lower pH) will cause the bicarbonate to gobble up some of the H$^+$ (lowering the concentration of HCO$_3^-$), leading to the generation of more carbonic acid, which can then dissociate into CO$_2$ and water. The CO$_2$ gas can be exhaled, thus reducing the effect of having added hydrogen ions.

Anion gap

The addition of many acids will increase the anion gap. Recognizing there must always be electroneutrality, if we add up all the cations (Na$^+$, K$^+$, Ca^{2+}, Mg^{2+}), they must equal all the anions (HCO$_3^-$, Cl$^-$, PO$_4^{3-}$, SO$_4^{3-}$, proteins, organic acids). Since we do not routinely measure the proteins and organic acids, these become the "anion gap," the difference between cations and anions.[6] We simplify all this math by only counting sodium, chloride, and bicarbonate and accepting as normal an anion gap of 12 mEq/L +/− 4 mEq/L thus,

$$\text{Anion gap} = \text{Na}^+ - (\text{Cl}^- + \text{HCO}_3^-)$$

Buffers

Were it not for buffers in blood and tissue, any change in hydrogen ion concentration would cause large swings of pH. The buffers in blood (primarily hemoglobin) avidly sop up hydrogen ions, mitigating shifts in pH; therefore, a severely anemic patient will experience greater shifts in pH than a patient with normal hemoglobin values. When buffering proves insufficient and correcting a low cardiac output fails to help, we must treat a serious metabolic acidosis with the titration of bicarbonate. We calculate the initial dose[7] as

$$\frac{0.3 \times \text{wt (kg)} \times (24 \, \text{mEq/L} - \text{actual HCO}_3^-)}{2}$$

which should not fully correct the acidemia. We then look at repeated blood gas values presenting pH, bicarbonate, and PCO_2, realizing that the addition of bicarbonate will increase the pH while also liberating CO_2, which must (if possible) be exhaled.

ABG interpretation

A normal room air[8] arterial blood gas in a nonpregnant[9] patient should look something like:

pH 7.35−7.45, PCO_2 35−45 mmHg, PO_2 75−100 mmHg,

HCO_3^- 22−26 mmol/L.

Other values include methemoglobin (met Hb) $<2\%$, carboxyhemoglobin (CO Hb) $<3\%$, and base excess −2 to 2 mEq/L.

When the laboratory reports abnormal results, we ask several questions:

(i) Is the PO_2 OK? Apply alveolar air equation.

(ii) Is the pH OK? If not, is there a metabolic or respiratory disturbance with or without compensation or is it a mixed disturbance? (See Table 10.3.)

Two clinical examples

Case 1: A PACU nurse calls because a post-operative patient has a low SpO_2, which did not normalize by giving the patient oxygen by face mask.

The findings:

(i) SpO_2 of 90% on FiO_2 of 0.5.

The alveolar air equation estimates (presuming – probably falsely – a normal arterial CO_2 of 40 mmHg) an alveolar oxygen tension of 306 mmHg (0.50 × (760−47) − (40/0.8)). A SpO_2 of 90% corresponds to a PaO_2 of approximately 60 mmHg. Thus there is a *large* A-a difference.

(ii) ABG: pH 7.28, PCO_2 55 mmHg, PO_2 60 mmHg, HCO_3^- 26 mmol/L.

The measured PaO_2 corresponds (miraculously exactly) with the estimated PaO_2 using the SpO_2 data. The elevated $PaCO_2$ of 55 mmHg indicates hypoventilation, which would explain the low PaO_2.

Step 1: The pH of 7.28 indicates acidemia.

Step 2: The elevated arterial carbon dioxide tension implies a respiratory source.

Step 3: The CO_2 is increased (55−40 = 15 mmHg). The pH fall of 0.12 (7.40−7.28) is consistent with an acute respiratory acidosis (0.08 per 10 mmHg rise in the CO_2). In confirmation, according to Table 10.2, an acute elevation of PCO_2 by 15 mmHg should be associated with a rise of bicarbonate of 1.5 mEq/L.

Table 10.3. Interpretation of acid-base disorders from an arterial blood gas analysis

1. Is the pH low (acidemia < 7.35) or high (alkalemia > 7.45)?
2. Compare the pH with the PCO_2 and HCO_3^-:

   Acidemia: $PaCO_2$ > 45 mmHg = respiratory

               $[HCO_3^-]$ < 20 mmol/L = metabolic

   Alkalemia: $PaCO_2$ <35 mmHg = respiratory

               $[HCO_3^-]$ > 28 mmol/L = metabolic
3. If the primary disturbance is respiratory, is it acute or chronic?

   Acute: pH changes 0.08 units per 10 mmHg change in $PaCO_2$

   Chronic: pH changes 0.03 units per 10 mmHg change in $PaCO_2$

   Confirm with the bicarbonate; it will not have had time to change much in an acute disturbance (Table 10.2).
4. If the primary disturbance is metabolic, is the respiratory response appropriate?

   Acidemia: $PaCO_2 = (1.5 \times HCO_3^-) + 8 (\pm 2)$ mmHg

   Alkalemia: $PaCO_2 = (0.7 \times HCO_3^-) + 21 (\pm 1.5)$ mmHg

   If the $PaCO_2$ is higher than expected, there is a coexisting primary respiratory acidosis; if lower, there is a respiratory alkalosis.
5. If there is a metabolic acidosis, is the anion gap > 12?

   $AG = [Na^+] - ([Cl^-] + [HCO_3^-])$
6. Consider the differential diagnosis for the resulting disorder(s) (see Table 10.4 for a representative (non-exhaustive) list).

The patient's bicarbonate confirms our suspicion that we are dealing with an acute, i.e., so far uncompensated, respiratory acidemia.

We must now determine whether obstruction (is the airway patent? Do bandages impede ventilation?), weakness (is there a muscle relaxant hangover?), or central depression (effects of narcotics?) can explain the hypoventilation. Therapy will depend on what we find.

Case 2: The ambulance brings a trauma patient to the Emergency Department. The patient has a fractured hip. As a routine, a nurse applies a face mask delivering 50% oxygen. SpO_2 is 100%. An ABG reveals: pH 7.23, PCO_2 25 mmHg, PO_2 250 mmHg, HCO_3^- 12 mmol/L.

(i) We welcome the SpO_2 of 100% but realize that the patient can still have a ventilation/perfusion abnormality. However, the PaO_2 of 250 mmHg confirms a small A-a difference ($PAO_2 = 0.5 \times (760-47) - 25/0.8 = 325$ mmHg).

(ii) *Step 1*: The pH of 7.23 shows acidemia.

     Step 2: The low $PaCO_2$ and HCO_3^- describe a metabolic source (with significant hyperventilation).

Table 10.4. Differential diagnosis of metabolic disorders (non-exhaustive list)

Anion gap metabolic acidosis: MUDPILERS

   M   Methanol*

   U   Uremia

   D   Diabetic or alcoholic ketoacidosis*

   P   Paraldehyde

   I   Iron, isoniazid, isopropyl alcohol*

   L   Lactic acidosis

   E   Ethylene glycol*, ethanol*

   R   Rhabdomyolysis

   S   Salicylates, strychnine

Non-anion gap metabolic acidosis

   Hyperchloremia (as with large-volume infusions of normal saline)

   Diarrhea

   Renal disease

   Carbonic anhydrase inhibitors

   Hyperalimentation

   Many others . . .

Metabolic alkalosis

   Emesis

   Administration of bicarbonate

*Often with an increased osmolar gap.

Step 3: The respiratory response is appropriate ($PCO_2 \approx 25 \approx (1.5 \times 12) +$ 8 mmHg).

We follow up with additional studies, such as electrolyte levels to calculate the anion gap, to identify the cause of the patient's trouble (Table 10.4).

Providing supplemental oxygen

If breathing room air, a patient's FiO_2 will be 0.21. FiO_2 is the *fraction* of inspired oxygen (0.21 at sea level as well as on Mount Everest) – frequently confused with the percentage of oxygen (21%) – frequently muddled with the partial pressure of oxygen (about 150 mmHg at sea level and much less on Mount Everest). We have several devices to increase the spontaneously breathing patient's FiO_2 (Fig. 10.5):

- Nasal cannula increases FiO_2 about 1–2% per liter (thus 2L delivers about 28% oxygen). Flow rates above 5 L irritate the nose without further increasing the FiO_2.

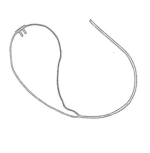 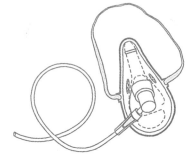 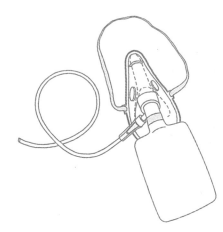

Fig. 10.5 Devices that provide supplemental oxygen. Nasal cannula (prongs), face mask, non-rebreather face mask.

- A loosely fitting oxygen mask with an oxygen flow rate of 6–8 L/min may bring the inspired oxygen percentage to 60–80%.
- A non-rebreathing face mask can deliver ~95% oxygen (the bag should be inflated . . . unlike what the flight attendants tell us).

For each device, we need an oxygen cylinder,[10] a reducing valve to bring the high pressure of a full cylinder to a manageable 40 psi (12 atm), and a flow meter that lets us select a flow rate anywhere from about 100 mL/min to 10 000 mL/min. The actual inspired concentration of oxygen will depend on the flow rate of oxygen, as well as the patient's peak inspiratory flow rate.

Pre-oxygenation/de-nitrogenation

Generally, tracheal intubation in adults is made easier with muscle relaxation, which causes apnea. An apneic healthy adult will begin to desaturate (decreasing oxyhemoglobin percentage, SpO_2) within 2 minutes. Young and healthy patients usually maintain close to 100% oxygen saturation while breathing room air. Increasing the inspired oxygen concentration will raise the arterial oxygen tension, but add relatively little to the overall oxygen content of blood, as explained above.

However, to provide a reservoir of oxygen in the lungs, we apply a tight-fitting mask and have the patient breathe 100% oxygen before inducing apnea. This reservoir occupies the functional residual capacity (FRC) of the lung (the volume remaining after normal exhalation, see Fig. 10.6). Notice that little of the total lung volume is actually exchanged with normal tidal ventilation; therefore, several minutes of pre-oxygenation, or four to five full vital capacity breaths, are required to maximize the oxygen depot in the FRC. Two requirements for effective denitrogenation: (i) we need to let the patient inhale pure oxygen, which

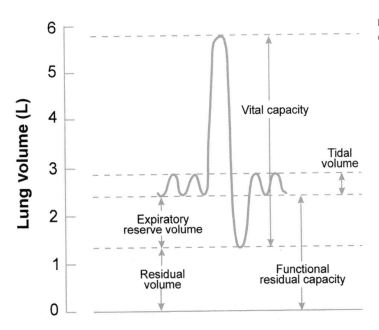

Fig. 10.6 Lung volumes and capacities

means the anesthesia machine must deliver at least a minute volume of oxygen to the patient in order to prevent the rebreathing of exhaled nitrogen (the carbon dioxide absorber takes care of the CO_2). (ii) The patient must ventilate his lungs long enough to wash out the nitrogen in the lungs. We usually think of this process in terms of time constants, that is to say that it will take about four time constants to approach near complete denitrogenation of the lungs (there will still be nitrogen in solution in the body). One time constant is the time required to deliver a volume of gas equal to the volume of the lungs. After one time constant, we will have replaced 63% of the gas in the lungs (with additional time constants we get to 86.5%, 95.0%, 98.2% and 99%, respectively). In a healthy, non-obese adult, with adequate pre-oxygenation (end-tidal oxygen concentration of >85%), this reservoir will provide 5–8 minutes of oxygen before the apneic patient's blood begins to desaturate.

Some factors can increase the rate of desaturation:
- A smaller reservoir: decreased FRC as in obesity, pregnancy, infancy.
- Increased oxygen consumption: hyperthermia, obesity, pregnancy, infancy.

Mechanical ventilation

Many patients require mechanical ventilation in the operating room or intensive care unit. While an intubated patient can breathe spontaneously through an endotracheal tube (which imposes significant resistance), many operative procedures require muscle relaxation, making mechanical ventilation mandatory. Most anesthesia machines are equipped with ventilators capable of providing volume- or pressure-controlled ventilation. For volume-controlled ventilation, the operator sets a tidal volume, respiratory rate, and inspiratory to expiratory time ratio ($I:E$ ratio), and the ventilator does its best to comply. If compliance deteriorates, the machine will generate additional pressure (up to a set limit) in an attempt to deliver the desired tidal volume. In pressure-controlled mode, as the name suggests, the selected pressure will be maintained for a set time, which might mean variable tidal volumes, depending on the patient's pulmonary compliance and resistance.

In general, ventilators used in the ICU offer more options than anesthesia machine ventilators. For example, they might offer SIMV (synchronized intermittent mandatory ventilation) in which the mechanical breath is synchronized with the patient's inspiratory effort, and the patient can breathe spontaneously between mechanical breaths. SIMV is often combined with pressure support ventilation (PSV), in which spontaneous respiratory efforts are met with a set level of positive pressure, assisting with inhalation and designed to overcome the resistance imposed by the endotracheal tube and ventilator.

Another ventilator mode that requires explanation is continuous positive airway pressure (CPAP) and positive end-expiratory pressure (PEEP). Ordinarily, when we exhale, some gas remains in the lungs (the FRC – see Fig. 10.6). Supine positioning and anesthesia reduce the FRC, potentially resulting in hypoxemia. Normal FRC can be restored with the addition of end-expiratory pressure, PEEP. It becomes particularly useful if increased intra-abdominal pressure or extravascular fluid (pulmonary edema, atelectasis, aspiration of gastric contents or respiratory distress syndrome (ARDS)) decreased FRC or caused collapse of alveoli. Two major factors limit the amount of PEEP that we can apply: (i) the increase in intrathoracic pressure will impede venous return; and (ii) the inspired tidal volume is administered on top of this baseline positive pressure, causing increased peak inflation pressure and possibly barotrauma.

Anesthesia in the patient with pulmonary disease

Patients with lung disease arrive at respiratory patterns optimal for their condition. This can include the recruitment of auxiliary muscles, changes in inspiratory and expiratory flow rates, respiratory rate, and arterial carbon dioxide tension. Because anesthesia can disturb these delicate adjustments, many anesthesiologists prefer to resort to regional anesthesia, where practical. Two major issues must be considered, however:

(i) The potential respiratory effects of the intended regional anesthetic. For example, a thoracic-level epidural anesthetic block begins to compromise intercostal muscle activity, reduces FRC, limits the patient's ability to cough, and theoretically can stimulate bronchospasm by blocking dilatory sympathetic innervation to the bronchi. Some approaches to the brachial plexus have a high incidence of unilateral phrenic nerve paralysis and an occasional pneumothorax. While the average patient can tolerate the loss of intercostal muscles, a "pulmonary cripple," who at rest uses accessory muscles to breathe, might be left with inadequate respiratory muscle strength.

(ii) The respiratory depressant effects of sedative medications might be accentuated in these patients. While it is preferable to attempt an anesthetic that avoids airway instrumentation, this preference turns into a liability if the need for emergent tracheal intubation arises should the patient slip into respiratory failure.

Asthma

The patient with well-controlled asthma should sail through general anesthesia without much difficulty. All asthma medications, and particularly steroids, should be continued pre-operatively. Nebulized albuterol (or another β_2 agonist) administered in the pre-operative holding area provides bronchodilation just before anesthesia. Because instrumentation of the airway can stimulate bronchospasm, patients with refractory asthma might benefit from anesthetic techniques that avoid airway manipulation, such as regional or local anesthesia with gentle intravenous sedation. Should general anesthesia be required, several options for induction and airway management are available. Small doses of either thiopental or propofol can ease the patient to sleep, at which point one of the halogenated inhalation anesthetics can be slowly introduced. These agents are bronchodilators. Ketamine is a bronchodilator as well and may be used, provided its potential side effects can be accepted. A laryngeal mask airway (LMA) is a lesser stimulus to bronchospasm than an endotracheal tube. When tracheal intubation becomes necessary, the goal at induction will be to completely block the airway reflexes that stimulate bronchospasm. Intravenous lidocaine (0.5–1.0 mg/kg) can prove helpful. Intravenous opioids (but not morphine which tends to release histamine) can be used. But remember that some patients develop respiratory difficulties (a "stiff chest") in response to large doses of opioids, the treatment of which requires muscle relaxation.

Intra-operatively, warm and humidified gases can reduce bronchospasm. Mechanical ventilation requires consideration of the pulmonary pathology. Asthmatics have a prolonged expiratory phase. If we do not give them enough time for exhalation, they will trap air ("dynamic hyperinflation"), resulting in increased intrathoracic pressures. This "auto-PEEP" reduces venous return and cardiac output. A prolonged expiratory time allows for full exhalation. Simply lengthening the exhalation time steals time from inhalation, which in turn might require high inspiratory pressures (the same tidal volume must be given over a shorter time).

Reducing the tidal volume and/or respiratory rate would help, but will necessarily reduce minute ventilation and entail the potential for hypercarbia. "Permissive hypercapnea" can become necessary when minute ventilation cannot be maintained without risk of barotrauma (pneumothorax).

Because stimulation of the trachea can trigger bronchospasm, removal of the endotracheal tube may be best accomplished during deep anesthesia. This is only appropriate in patients at low risk for aspiration and obstruction of the upper airway. Prophylactic supplemental oxygen in the post-operative period can prevent hypoxia-induced airway reactivity.

Obstructive sleep apnea

Obstructive sleep apnea (OSA) occurs when the soft tissues of the pharynx collapse during sleep, obstructing the airway and resulting in hypoxemia. Sleep apnea plagues obese patients who snore heavily with intermittent bouts of obstruction to the point of apnea (reported by partner) and repeated awakening. During the day, they are often somnolent. The apneic periods cause hypoxemia and hypercarbia, resulting in (i) cardiac irritability with bradycardia and premature ventricular contractions (PVCs), (ii) vasoconstriction, both peripherally (leading to increased systemic vascular resistance and hypertension) and in the pulmonary circulation (with pulmonary hypertension and potentially right heart failure), and (iii) erythropoeisis (resulting in polycythemia). Because of the potential of thrombosis and unfavorable rheology, a polycythemic patient should be phlebotomized if the hematocrit is too high (>55%).

Should you obtain a history of OSA during the anesthesia pre-operative evaluation, you may have to order further studies including ECG and possibly echocardiogram to look for evidence of pulmonary hypertension and right heart compromise. In a subset of patients ("Pickwickians"), ABG analysis might demonstrate daytime CO_2 retention with potentially impaired hypercarbic respiratory drive. Therapeutic interventions include nasal CPAP during sleep, weight loss, and surgical correction. OSA patients are particularly sensitive to opioids and sedatives and can develop airway obstruction with even low doses of respiratory depressants. Finally, patients with excess pharyngeal tissue and obesity present difficulties with airway management. Not only can intubation be tough, we may be unable to mask–ventilate or even use an LMA. Thus ventilation may be very difficult to provide once we render the patient unconscious and paralyzed.

Pulmonary problems during anesthesia

Once the airway is secured, many things can still go wrong with the pulmonary system. Often – but not invariably – pulse oximetry gives the first signal of trouble:

(i) We have to provide oxygen into the airway. Problems arise when (inadvertently) another gas is substituted for oxygen, or when a mechanical problem affects the delivery mechanism (like failure to turn on the ventilator or a disconnection of the ventilator from the breathing circuit).

(ii) We need to have adequate alveolar ventilation, i.e., tidal volumes in excess of deadspace. Problems include a kinked or plugged ETT, a leak somewhere (allowing the gas to vent to the atmosphere), bronchospasm, pneumothorax, a plug (mucus, blood, tissue, foreign body) in a bronchus, decreased lung compliance, increased intrathoracic pressure (as with insufflation of carbon dioxide into the abdomen for laparoscopy), inadequate fresh gas flow rate, or increased apparatus deadspace as from machine valve failure.

(iii) When the oxygen arrives at the alveolus, it has to be able to get into the blood stream. Problems here include a diffusion block in the alveolus (pulmonary edema fluid), lack of blood flow to the alveolus (pulmonary embolism), or inability of the blood to pick up oxygen, e.g., carbon monoxide poisoning – though this would fool the SpO_2 into reporting normal saturation; see Monitoring chapter).

(iv) Finally, the oxygenated blood has to make it to the location of the pulse oximeter for analysis. Problems here would include dilution of the oxygenated blood with venous blood (shunt), flow blockade to the location of the pulse oximeter (distal to an inflated blood pressure cuff or tourniquet), presence of dyes that can alter the color of the blood (methylene blue), inaccurate probe placement (only partially on the finger), or failure of the oximeter probe itself.

So, in addition to calling for help . . .

(i) Check FiO_2 (if unexpectedly low, disconnect from wall oxygen source and use oxygen from a cylinder or room air).

(ii) Increase FiO_2, e.g., turn off nitrous oxide, increase fresh gas flow with oxygen.

(iii) Check capnogram shape of $ETCO_2$ waveform – in short, confirm adequate gas exchange.

(iv) Check pulse oximeter waveform and probe (reposition as needed).

(v) Listen to breath sounds bilaterally – mainstem intubation? Pneumothorax? Inadvertent extubation?

(vi) Check peak inspiratory pressure – if low, there may be a leak; if high, an obstruction.

   (a) Give several manual breaths – while it turns out that even "educated hands" cannot gauge compliance and resistance well, a few slow, deep manual breaths allow control over the pattern of inspiration, which may improve the situation. However, we must be careful not to get stuck just squeezing the bag to feel as if we are doing something, tying up our hands when we could be handling other needs. Also, anesthesia machines and ventilators will generate peak inspiratory pressure and tidal volume *data* (rather than impressions). Observing these two parameters during anesthesia helps us detect trends that might herald problems before they become emergencies.

(b) Suction ETT – confirms patency and removes secretions.

(vii) Check exhaled tidal volume (to ensure there is no leak).

(viii) Consider obtaining arterial blood gases and chest radiograph.

(ix) PEEP – administering PEEP may improve the saturation, since often the cause is decreased FRC. Inspiratory pressures and/or venous return can constrain the level of PEEP.

NOTES

1. In the presence of oxygen, cells metabolize glucose through the Krebs cycle and electron transport chain, netting 36 ATP. Without oxygen, glycolysis proceeds, but nets only 2 ATP and a bunch of lactic acid.

2. Adolph Eugen Fick (1829–1901), a German physician, physiologist and physicist. He came up with this diffusion equation when just 26 years old! He is even more famous for describing the calculation of cardiac output still in use today (cardiac output = oxygen consumption / arterial-venous oxygen content difference).

3. $D = \dfrac{S}{\sqrt{MW}}$; S = solubility, MW = molecular weight.

4. $P_AO_2 = P_IO_2 - P_ACO_2 \times [FiO_2 + (1 - FiO_2)/R]$, which corrects for the fact that an $R < 1$ results in a lower volume of exhaled gas.

5. Lawrence Joseph Henderson (1878–1942) linked [H^+] and buffers as [H^+] = Ka([acid]/[salt]); later Karl Albert Hasselbalch (1874–1962) coupled this with Søren Sørensen's pH scale to produce the now famous equation: pH = pKa + log ([A^-]/[HA]).

6. Albumin contributes the most to the gap. A fall in albumin concentration by 1 gram lowers the anion gap by 2.5–3 mmol/L. Thus hypoalbuminemia must be considered when calculating the anion gap.

7. This equation determines the missing bicarbonate (normal – actual), and its normal distribution in the extracellular fluid (0.3 × body weight in kg), then replaces only 1/2 that amount.

8. It is common to specify "room" air which, when dry, contains 20.947% oxygen, 78.084% nitrogen, 0.934% argon and 0.033% carbon dioxide. The rest is made up of – in decreasing concentrations – neon, helium, krypton, sulfur dioxide, methane, hydrogen, nitrous oxide, xenon, ozone, nitrogen dioxide, iodine, carbon monoxide and ammonia. Medical compressed air often contains a little more carbon dioxide (up to 0.05%) than room air and trace amounts of oil (up to 0.5 g per cubic meter). Clinically these differences can be ignored.

9. Pregnant women normally bring their arterial blood gas to pH 7.44, $PaCO_2$ 30 mmHg, HCO_3^- 20 mEq/L. This must be taken into account when interpreting a maternal ABG.

10. Oxygen cylinders contain gaseous oxygen under pressure to 2000 psi (pounds per square inch) or 600 atm. They are painted green in the US and white in much of Europe.

11

Anesthesia and other systems

If you are reading this, you are not a neurologist, gastroenterologist, hepatologist, nephrologist, or hematologist. Yet, anesthesiologists need to worry about some features and functions of the stomach, liver, kidneys, blood, and particularly the brain. Here is a short perspective on the why and how.

The brain

General anesthesia is, ultimately, about putting the central nervous system (CNS) to sleep. We choose this or that agent in an effort to optimize the patient's intraoperative course, but in reality the nuances of the different agents make little difference a few days after minor surgery in a healthy patient. However, in the patient with intracranial pathology, a thorough understanding of neurophysiology and the implications of anesthesia take center stage. Because we do not know which patients have undiagnosed cerebral aneurysms or tumors, we like to apply our understanding to all patients.

The brain is an amazing organ. Despite weighing only about 1.3 kg, just 2% of total body weight, it receives 15% of the cardiac output and consumes 20% of the oxygen used by the body and watches over all of the body! Formulating some mental models of this metabolic workhorse will help to explain its dynamic workings. Conveniently, the spinal cord behaves physiologically similar to the brain.

Compared to other organs, cerebral hemodynamics have both similarities and unique features. Numerous factors affect the cerebral vascular system (Table 11.1). The brain autoregulates cerebral blood flow (CBF) to maintain it stable at cerebral perfusion pressures (CPP) between 65 mmHg and 150 mmHg. But similar to virtually all other organs, it also couples flow to metabolism to assure active areas of the brain receive enough oxygen and glucose to sustain their activities. The cerebral vascular network, curiously, has few alpha-1 receptors. This makes phenylepherine a preferred choice for correcting hypotension without constriction cerebral vessels. Opposite to the pulmonary artery's response, brain vascular

Table 11.1. Effect of systemic and local factors on cerebrovascular resistance

Cerebral vasoconstriction is observed with:
Increased blood pressure (autoregulation)
Hyperoxia (PaO_2 > 300 mmHg produces 12% decrease of CBF)
Decreased $PaCO_2$ (every 1 mmHg reduction in $PaCO_2$ decreases CBF 4%)
Decreased blood viscosity
Decreased cerebral metabolic demands
    Barbiturates (decrease CBF up to 60% by producing isoelectric EEG)
    Lowered temperature

Cerebral vasodilatation is observed with:
Decreased blood pressure (autoregulation)
Increased $PaCO_2$
Increased blood viscosity
Hypoxia (PaO_2 < 60 mmHg)
Increased cerebral metabolic demands
    Stress state
    Fever
Vessels surrounding brain tumors lose CO_2 responsiveness and remain maximally
    dilated.

responsiveness to hypercarbia causes vasodilatation while hypocarbia produces vasoconstriction and, in extreme cases, can produce cerebral ischemia.

The skull rigidly constrains the volume of the intracranial space and its three constituents: brain tissue (1100 g or mL), blood (75 mL), and cerebrospinal fluid (150 mL). The falx cerebri divides the brain into a left and right hemisphere, while the tentorium cerebelli separates the cerebellum from the rest. If any of the brain components increases in volume, either the others must shrink by a similar amount, or the intracranial pressure (ICP) increases (Fig. 11.1). This increased pressure may manifest as papilledema on fundoscopic examination, and as narrowed ventricles or midline shift on an imaging study. Clinical signs include nausea, vomiting, ataxia, altered mental status or the seldom seen Cushing's triad[1] of bradycardia, hypertension and bradypnea.

Intracranial hypertension poses a significant threat. As the intracranial pressure (ICP) increases beyond a critical point, blood flow to the brain decreases. However, the brain has no stored oxygen. It withstands limited ischemic exposures only by increasing its blood flow or increasing its oxygen extraction from hemoglobin. The brain is a metabolic engine that uses only glucose (or ketones) and oxygen for energy. Sixty percent of the energy used by the brain is spent on performing electrophysiologic functions and 40% on preserving cellular integrity. Thus, defending cerebral perfusion and oxygen delivery are intrinsic to the management

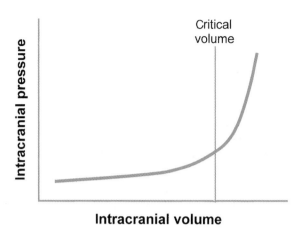

Critical
volume

Intracranial pressure

Intracranial volume

Fig. 11.1 Intracranial pressure
with increasing intracranial
volume.

of all intracranial masses and elevated ICP. As with all organs, perfusion depends
on the pressure difference across the organ:

$$CPP = MAP - CVP \text{ or } ICP$$

where CPP is cerebral perfusion pressure; MAP, mean arterial pressure; CVP,
central venous pressure; ICP, intracranial pressure (normal mean <15 mmHg).
Thus CPP depends on both arterial blood pressure, and the higher of CVP or ICP.

When intracranial hypertension continues to rise, the increasing pressure on
the brain must eventually "pop off" into another area. This spontaneous decom-
pression is termed "herniation" and can occur via transtentorial, uncal, subfal-
cine, across the foramen magnum (tonsillar) or out of the skull, when a fracture
offers an opening. Tonsillar herniation pushes the brainstem through the foramen magnum, a life-threatening emergency. Herniation is a critical event, not
simply because of the implications of local ischemia – from which a recovery may
be possible – but also because with herniation, sheer forces produce irreparable
mechanical disruption.

With general anesthesia, we aim to produce a sleeping, well perfused and oxygenated brain. Unfortunately, we possess little information about what is actually
happening in the brain and are left with doing our best by using our understanding of how the seat of the soul works. For example, we know that the EEG
begins to demonstrate an ischemic pattern when the CBF decreases below about
20 mL/100 g brain/min, a reduction of over 50% from its normal 50 mL/100 g
brain/min perfusion. Hence, hypotension must be treated even in the absence of
cardiac ischemia.

In the presence of intracranial pathology, we intentionally address each of the
intracerebral volumes to optimize the intra-operative course. We lower the blood
volume by placing the patient in a slightly head-up position to facilitate venous
drainage. Barbiturates given for induction cause an isoelectric EEG (always, but

Table 11.2. Methods to reduce intracranial pressure

- Hyperventilation – in the short term, hyperventilation to an arterial PCO_2 of 25 mmHg can reduce cerebral blood flow, reducing ICP. This must be balanced, however, against the increased intrathoracic pressure required to hyperventilate the patient's lungs, which can reduce venous return causing hypotension. Also, vasoconstriction in the areas under carbon dioxide control might decrease compensatory blood flow.
- Mannitol – bolus administration of this 6-carbon sugar has two effects: (i) it expands the blood volume and decreases viscosity, improving cerebral blood flow; and (ii) it generates an osmotic gradient in the brain, drawing water out of brain tissue. The net effect – an acute reduction in ICP. However, the subsequent diuresis can exacerbate hypovolemia, and in the presence of poor renal perfusion the high osmolality can trigger acute tubular necrosis.
- Elevating the head of the bed to about 30° – this simple maneuver can reduce ICP, but can also impair venous return from the lower extremities. Trauma patients are often placed in Trendelenburg position (with the head below the level of the legs) to increase venous return, a maneuver best avoided in patients with high ICP.
- Fluid management – hypotonic solutions and those containing glucose clearly worsen neurologic outcome by encouraging brain swelling. With an intact blood brain barrier, hypertonic solutions might provide an advantage by *reducing* brain swelling.
- Glucocorticoids – reduce edema associated with brain tumors and are also indicated for the treatment of acute spinal cord injury; but steroids do not reduce edema from traumatic brain injuries.
- Hypothermia – brings the advantage of reduced oxygen consumption (in the absence of shivering, basal metabolic rate falls by 7% per 1 °C of temperature reduction). But hypothermia raises other problems: the patient might shiver which dramatically raises oxygen consumption, coagulation is profoundly disturbed which can worsen intracerebral hemorrhage and arrhythmias can be triggered with temperatures below 30 °C.
- Barbiturate coma – reserved for the most severely injured who have failed to respond to more conservative therapy. High barbiturate plasma levels reduce cerebral metabolic rate and cerebral blood flow thus lowering ICP until the injury can heal. Unfortunately, barbiturates depress the cardiovascular system.
- CSF drainage – after a ventriculostomy has been placed, we can readily reduce the CSF volume. Draining CSF from a lumbar tap, however, can result in herniation of the brain in the foramen magnum in the presence of brain swelling and elevated ICP. Hence the admonition to look for clinical signs and symptoms of elevated ICP before performing a lumbar puncture or neuraxial anesthetic.

only briefly at standard doses) and a subsequent autoregulated decrease in CBF. We usually avoid ketamine and halothane because they increase CBF and dramatically increase ICP. We may induce mild hyperventilation to produce arterial vasoconstriction. Under specific circumstances, we might have to remove CSF peri-operatively via a ventriculostomy or spinal drain. In the presence of edema or a large mass, we might use steroids and diuretics to reduce the interstitial volume and, through oxygen free radical scavenging, protect the brain from ischemic insult. Should the ICP be high, we must defend CPP, for example by increasing the mean arterial pressure with phenylepherine.

An aneurysm or arteriovenous malformation challenges us to maintain stable pressures across the vascular wall by balancing the ICP against the MAP. We might lower temperature when we anticipate regional ischemic events as can

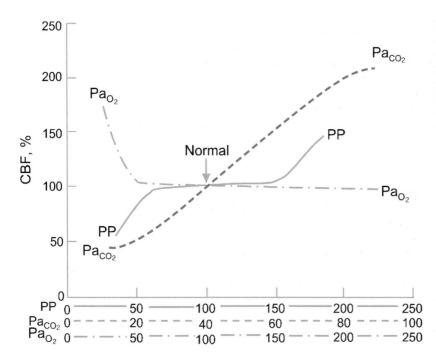

Fig. 11.2 Cerebral blood flow in a changing environment. Cerebral blood flow (CBF) responds to changes in perfusion pressure (PP = MAP − (ICP or CVP)), as well as arterial oxygen (PaO_2) and carbon dioxide ($PaCO_2$) tensions. MAP: mean arterial pressure; ICP: intracranial pressure; CVP: central venous pressure.

occur when temporary clips are placed to facilitate definitive aneurysm clipping. Otherwise, we work to keep patients warm. The potent inhalational anesthetics all uncouple metabolism-flow autoregulation, causing a decreased metabolic rate but increasing the CBF. Hence, we use the halogenated vapors in modest concentrations during intracranial surgery.

Consider how one might approach a trauma patient with both arterial hypotension and increased ICP from a subdural hematoma (SDH). We will work feverishly to increase his MAP but must also strive to reduce ICP (Table 11.2). We treat low blood pressure in a trauma patient with the infusion of fluids and, as mentioned above, intravenous phenylepherine. In addition to CPP, arterial oxygen and carbon dioxide tensions affect cerebral blood flow and therefore ICP (Fig. 11.2). We might acutely manipulate $PaCO_2$ in an effort to reduce ICP in the short term; however, aggressive hyperventilation to decrease ICP can worsen outcome, probably because it can decrease CBF.

Until the last decade of the twentieth century, the brain remained an organ that could not be easily monitored. We had to be guided by changes in heart rate, blood pressure, urine output, and the patient's motor response. Today, we monitor raw and processed EEG, e.g., BIS® monitoring, Aspect Medical, to aid us in titrating our drugs, avoiding and treating cerebral ischemia and reducing intra-operative awareness.

The stomach

The stomach should be empty before we give general anesthesia because regurgitating or vomiting and then, because of obtunded reflexes, inhaling the stuff found in the stomach can lead to serious trouble. The aspirated particulate matter can lodge in a distal bronchus, get infected, and result in bronchopneumonia or lung abscess. A large particle can block a mainstem bronchus or the trachea with obvious dire consequences. Even in the OR, a patient can be treated with the Heimlich maneuver. Given an unconscious patient and the worry about more regurgitation and aspiration, tools such as a bronchoscope and suction available in the OR might be better suited for retrieval of foreign matter in the trachea or upper bronchial tree.

More common than particulate aspiration is the aspiration of gastric juice. If it has a pH under 2.5 and a volume of more than 0.4–1.0 mL/kg, the aspirate can cause the infamous Mendelson syndrome, a nasty chemical burn of the lungs that can be fatal. Treatment consists of support of ventilation, often with positive end expiratory pressure (PEEP) in order to expand the bronchioles and alveoli, reduce edema, and improve gas exchange.

The potential of gastric acid aspiration leads us to take precautions. The idea of emptying the stomach with help of a gastric tube comes to mind. While it might decompress a full stomach by removing gas and liquid, it cannot empty the stomach and is rather unkind in the awake patient. For elective surgery, we ask patients to take nothing by mouth for several hours before anesthesia. We also have drugs available to increase gastric pH and reduce volume as indicated. Even with such appropriate preparations, for patients with a full stomach or gastroesophageal reflux disease (GERD), we would resort to a rapid sequence induction (see General anesthesia).

The liver

We expect this large organ to do its biotransformation magic on many of the drugs we give. For example, the liver avidly removes propofol, which is said to have a hepatic extraction ratio (HER) of close to 1. Reduced liver blood flow will, therefore, reduce the rate of propofol biotransformation. The rate of biotransformation of drugs with a low HER, such as thiopental, will be less affected by changes in liver blood flow. Remember that the liver normally receives about 25% of cardiac output, roughly 2/3 of that via the low-pressure portal system, the rest by way of the hepatic artery delivering oxygenated blood. General anesthesia tends to reduce cardiac output and, proportionally, hepatic arterial blood flow more than portal blood flow. The hepatic circulation is also richly supplied with alpha receptors; hence the administration of alpha active vasopressors will reduce hepatic blood flow. Because of the enormous reserves of the liver, we rarely see the consequences of reduced liver blood supply. Even in the face of mild to moderate hepatic failure, the liver attends to its biotransformation job. There are limits to what even the most faithful of livers can accomplish.

Liver enzymes

The liver attacks many drugs with mixed function oxidases of which the cytochrome P-450 system represents a well-known member. In this first phase of hepatic biotransformation, drugs may be degraded to ineffective compounds (for example, the benzodiazepines and barbiturates) or to active substances (for example, meperidine becomes normeperidine). In the second phase, drugs undergo conjugation, often leading to more water-soluble compounds prepared for renal elimination.

When drugs such as ethanol or barbiturates stimulate the production of enzymes, we speak of enzyme induction, which often affects the P-450 system. With more enzyme available, the biotransformation of some drugs will be accelerated, leading to greater tolerance and reduced drug effect. Some drugs, such as cimetidine, can inhibit the P-450 system and thus enhance the effect of drugs dependent on the system's detoxifying activity.

Liver function studies

We assess liver function by searching for liver enzymes spilled into the blood. We often ask the simple question: is the patient's hepatic disease brought about by biliary obstruction (elevated bilirubin and alkaline phosphatase) or hepatocellular dysfunction (prolonged prothrombin time, low plasma albumin and elevated SGOT and SGPT)?[2]

Halothane hepatitis

Soon after halothane was introduced in the late 1950s, concerns arose about a new entity called halothane hepatitis. Several case reports described sometimes fatal acute hepatitis in patients exposed to the drug. In the meantime, other halogenated anesthetics have also been implicated. Suspicion was directed at the potentially toxic effects of the products of biotransformation of the halogenated vapors, particularly if they arose during hypoxic conditions. Because patients repeatedly exposed to the drug appeared to have a higher incidence of "halothane hepatitis," a sensitivity reaction was suspected. However, uncounted patients had many repeated halothane anesthetics without ill effect. Many investigators believe that most cases of so-called halothane hepatitis have nothing to do with the anesthetic agent and are instead evidence of a post-operative recrudescence of viral hepatitis. Others think that the products of anaerobic biotransformation, particularly those involving fluoride (trifluoroacetic acid), can cause trouble in sensitive patients.

The kidneys

The kidneys concern us when drugs or their products of biotransformation need to be eliminated in urine. For this route out of the body, the substances need to be non-protein-bound so that they make it through the glomeruli and are then ionized so as to escape tubular reabsorption.

Impaired renal function becomes relevant with advancing years (creatinine clearance declines with age), with low cardiac output and decreased glomerular filtration, and with renal disease. The elimination of some drugs can be affected by decreased renal function. Of greatest interest to the anesthesiologist are a number of muscle relaxants such as pancuronium and doxacurium and their antagonist, neostigmine. Thus for patients in renal failure, we might elect atracurium or cisatracurium, muscle relaxants that undergo hydrolysis in plasma making them independent of renal excretion.

Patients in renal failure present special challenges not only because they cannot eliminate drugs in urine, but also because their water and electrolyte balance goes through roller coaster swings with intermittent dialysis. Ideally, the patient should have undergone dialysis within 24 hours before the anesthetic. Intra-operatively, the intravenous fluids need to be managed carefully, as the patient has no mechanism to eliminate excess water or electrolytes. These patients tend to be anemic with a reduced oxygen-carrying capacity, which puts an extra burden on the heart should it be called on to increase cardiac output in order to compensate for reduced delivery of oxygen to the tissues. Vascular access is often a problem in patients with arteriovenous fistulas.

In patients at risk of major changes of renal perfusion (operations with anticipated great blood loss, cardiac insufficiency, vascular procedures affecting renal blood flow or ureteral function), we often monitor urine production by collecting urine with the help of an indwelling urinary catheter (Foley). The gold standard of normal function calls for urine flow of around 0.5 ml/kg/h, though renal failure may occur at even higher rates of urine output, and often enough, patients make less urine intra-operatively without sliding into acute renal failure or tubular necrosis. After all, complex physiologic mechanisms enable the kidney to reduce urine production and to conserve blood volume. ADH (antidiuretic hormone, also known as vasopressin), whose job it is to retain fluid in the face of hypovolemia, is secreted during anesthesia even without the normal triggers. Regardless, if fluid deficits cannot account for reduced urine production, and there is no reason to assume reduced kidney blood flow e.g., secondary to hypotension, low cardiac output or because of mechanical interference with renal blood flow, and we confirm the Foley catheter is intact (not kinked or compressed), we begin to worry about acute tubular damage, for which a number of direct or indirect acting toxins (including antibiotics, chemotherapeutic agents and contrast dyes) can be responsible. Acute tubular damage, if not too severe, can undergo spontaneous repair over days to weeks.

The blood

Three functions of the blood demand attention: its volume, its oxygen-carrying capacity, and its ability or propensity to clot.

Volume

Blood volume varies with age, weight, and sex (see Vascular access and fluid management). As we know from donating blood, the average adult can easily lose 500 mL without conspicuous consequences. Indeed, healthy patients can tolerate a blood loss of 20% of their total blood volume. The body compensates for such loss by mobilizing interstitial and eventually even intracellular water to replenish the decreased intravascular volume. In the process, the hematocrit will fall gradually over a couple of days.

Oxygen-carrying capacity

With a loss of blood volume, the patient also loses oxygen carrying capacity. Compensatory increases in cardiac output can insure uninterrupted delivery of oxygen, even in the anemic patient. As hematocrit decreases to about 30%, fluidity of blood increases, which improves flow and thus aids in the delivery of a higher cardiac output. There are limits to how much anemia can be tolerated. If the anemia develops over weeks or months, astonishingly low hematocrit values can be compatible with an active life, though the patient will deal with easy fatigability. Thus, we cannot with confidence identify a certain hematocrit value that compels us to administer red cells. The idea that a hematocrit below 30% would lead us to administer packed cells has long been abandoned; even 18% is now often accepted. Instead of picking a threshold at which we would call for a transfusion, we take many factors into account. We might merely watch an anemic patient with a good cardiovascular system and normal CNS and renal function, while the same hematocrit in a patient with congestive failure and arrhythmias or confusion signals an urgent need to increase oxygen carrying capacity. Generally, we expect a single transfusion (450 mL packed cells) to increase the hematocrit by 3 volume % in the average adult.

Clotting

Like everything in life, too much of a good thing can be as bad as not enough. Thus, we find ourselves time and again in the position of interfering with the clotting mechanism to prevent thrombosis, or stimulating the system when the patient is at risk of bleeding into vital organs. In order to approach this problem in a rational manner, we need to recapitulate the normal clotting cascade. We will not delve into the details that fascinate hematologists and instead focus on specific points of common interest to anesthesiologists.

The normal clotting mechanism prevents uncounted (and unnoticed) bleeding opportunities in everyday life. This normal clotting mechanism is extraordinarily complex with a dizzying array of factors and steps, the most important to anesthesia being the following:

Platelets

Normally we have 150 000 to 450 000 platelets/μL. Surgical bleeding becomes a problem with counts below 50 000/μL, and spontaneous bleeding occurs below 20 000/μL. In patients with thrombocytopenia, we can increase the platelet count by 5000 to 10 000/μL with every platelet "pack," necessitating multiple units in most patients (order 1 unit/10 kg body weight). Platelets have a limited survival of up to 5 days if properly stored. Note that, unless specifically requested, platelets are "random donor pooled" meaning the patient is exposed to MANY donors at once with platelet transfusions. In contrast, one single donor unit is equivalent to about 6 units of pooled platelets.

Calcium

It plays a crucial role in the clotting cascade (where it is honored as factor IV). In stored blood, the calcium is bound up and deactivated by citrate. With massive (equivalent to an entire blood volume or more) and rapid blood transfusion, the liver may not be able to keep up the metabolism of calcium citrate, at which point plasma citrate can rise to the point where it will interfere with calcium's function as a coagulation factor. Citrate intoxication will also cause hypotension, cardiac depression, and prolonged QT intervals.

Congenital hemorrhagic diseases
- Von Willebrand's disease is the most common inherited bleeding disorder. It comes in different degrees of severity and is associated with a decreased or qualitatively abnormal von Willebrand's factor (VIII:vWF).
- Classic hemophilia (A), a genetic disease affecting males, is a factor VIII deficiency. Patients often suffer hemarthroses and have hematuria.
- Hemophilia B or Christmas Disease clinically resembles hemophilia A but is caused by a deficiency of factor IX.

Before anesthesia, these patients are treated with specific drugs, e.g., desmopressin (DDAVP[3®]) for von Willebrand's disease, or factor transfusion.

Heparin

The drug exhibits a medley of effects resulting in the inhibition of thrombin. Heparin is frequently given in the OR when coagulation must be stopped – as in vascular and cardiovascular procedures. In small doses, it is given to patients at risk for post-operative thrombosis. The effect of heparin is measured by the activated partial thromboplastin time (aPTT) and can be reversed by the administration of protamine, a highly positively charged molecule that binds the highly negatively charged heparin. Of note, the effect of low molecular weight heparins (LMWH, e.g., enoxaparin) cannot be assayed by aPTT (requires an anti-Factor Xa activity assay), and is not completely reversed by protamine.

Warfarin-type agents

These oral anticoagulants inhibit vitamin K-dependent factors (II, VII, IX, and X). Their activity is assayed by the prothrombin time (PT), with a therapeutic range of 1.5–4 times normal. These agents can be reversed by the administration of vitamin K, or acutely by transfusing fresh frozen plasma (FFP).

Coagulation studies

The coagulation status of a patient can be assessed clinically: is there evidence of bleeding (bloody urine, black stools (blood in upper GI tract), bleeding gums and/or easy bruising)? There are several laboratory tests to evaluate the clotting cascade.

Prothrombin time (PT)

This tests the extrinsic coagulation cascade and is prolonged when tissue factors are involved. Because there are differences between labs, an international normalized ratio (INR) has been adopted, with a normal value of 1.0.

Activated partial thromboplastin time (aPTT, normally 25–40 s)

This tests the intrinsic pathway of coagulation and almost all the factors except VII and XIII. We use this test to monitor heparin activity.

Activated clotting time (ACT, normally <120 s)

This is commonly used in the OR to test therapeutic heparin anticoagulation, e.g., during cardiopulmonary bypass or vascular surgery. We mix 2 mL of the patient's blood in a test tube containing an activator of coagulation, such as celite (diatomaceous earth), kaolin, or glass particles. We then stir the blood and monitor the time to clot formation. An ACT>200 s indicates adequate anticoagulation for these procedures. Note ACT is not a good monitor for lesser levels of heparin anticoagulation, e.g., deep venous thrombosis (DVT) prophylaxis.

The thromboelastogram (TEG)

This is used much less frequently. A clever machine scrutinizes the whole clotting process by analyzing the patient's blood in an oscillating cup as it clots around a piston. Developing fibrin between cup and piston transmits the oscillations, which are then recorded. As the clot forms, the device records the transmitted oscillations and, when normal, assume the shape of a bomb (no fins!). Abnormal clotting because of the presence of anticoagulants or thrombocytopenia or fibrinolysis causes the bomb to look spindly or skinny, or leaf-shaped. Cognoscenti can read these shapes like a book. If you are not in that league you can find details and pictures in: http://www.anest.ufl.edu/EA.

We detail replacement of clotting factors in Vascular access and fluid management.

NOTES

1. Harvey Williams Cushing (1869–1939), an American pioneer in neurosurgery, also lends his name to several syndromes with CNS pathology, a surgical clip and even an ulcer.
2. SGOT is serum glutamic-oxaloacetic transaminase also known as AST = serum aspartate aminotransaminase. SGPT is serum glutamic-pyruvic transaminase also known as ALT = serum alanine aminotransaminase.
3. DDAVP = 1-deamino-8-D-arginine vasopressin also known as desmopressin.

12

A brief pharmacology related to anesthesia

Approaching the anesthesia task with drugs

The basic approach

Many different approaches to general anesthesia are possible. Often, preoperative preparation includes the administration of drugs to (i) minimize the chance of aspiration of gastric juice, (ii) minimize anxiety and – if necessary – (iii) provide analgesia. Once the patient is in the operating room, we aim to denitrogenate the patient's lungs, followed by induction of anesthesia. One technique is to induce sleep with thiopental, give a paralyzing dose of succinylcholine to facilitate intubation of the trachea, and then maintain anesthesia with a halogenated anesthetic vapor administered together with nitrous oxide and, of course, oxygen. Muscle relaxation during the operation might be accomplished with one of the non-depolarizing neuromuscular blockers, frequently called "muscle relaxants." Another technique might start with propofol instead of thiopental and it might rely on large doses of an opiate, such as fentanyl and, to assure amnesia, a low concentration of a halogenated inhalation anesthetic. Many different combinations of these approaches are in use.

At the end of anesthesia and if the patient is still weakened from the muscle relaxant, the neuromuscular blockade has to be reversed with, for example, neostigmine given together with an anticholinergic drug. When the patient responds to commands, we remove the endotracheal tube and return the patient to the post-anesthesia care unit (PACU).

Drug interaction

The practice of anesthesia involves the administration of several drugs, some of them with overlapping effects. For example, premedication with midazolam (Versed®, a benzodiazepine) will make the patient more sensitive to the side effects of narcotic analgesics; neuromuscular blockade can be more readily achieved if the patient is in surgical anesthesia from a halogenated vapor than if anesthesia relies on nitrous oxide and narcotics. The degree of surgical stimulation will influence the patient's response to anesthetic drugs. During a small bowel anastomosis, which does not represent major noxious stimulation, less anesthesia will be required than when stimulating the carina with a suction catheter, for example. An elderly or debilitated or abstentious patient will require less depressant drug for the same effect than a young and vigorous person accustomed to regular alcohol intake. Drugs that undergo biotransformation with the help of enzymes that had been induced may have a shorter duration of action (some barbiturates) or more side effects, e.g., halothane biotransformation liberating hepatotoxins, than in the absence of induced enzymes. Repeated exposure to a drug can induce marked tolerance to the drug as is well known for narcotics. In other words, our brief discussion of pharmacology cannot cover all factors that might influence the patient's response to a cited dose.

In this chapter, we will look at the drugs typically used in anesthesia. First, however, a word about the theories of anesthesia.

Theories of anesthesia

Please note that we are speaking of theories (in the plural!). This simply reflects the fact that a single theory could not possibly explain the phenomenon of induced coma: there are simply too many different substances that can render a person reversibly unconscious. In some instances, we can imagine a mechanism, for example, lack of oxygen will stop the functioning of cells dependent on oxygen. But then think of a knock on the head, very high or low blood sugar, alcohol, sleeping pills, noble gases (xenon), inorganic gases (nitrous oxide), acetone, organic solvents such as chloroform, carbon tetrachloride, trichlorethylene, ethylene, diethyl ether, and a slew of halogenated compounds, not to mention narcotics, benzodiazepines, barbiturates, steroids, phenols, etc. To complicate matters, one fluorinated hydrocarbon, hexafluorodiethyl ether, is a convulsant (in the past used instead of electroconvulsant therapy in the treatment of depression) while several of its close relatives (isoflurane, enflurane, desflurane, sevoflurane) are in common use as anesthetics. Isoflurane and enflurane are isomers, both being di-fluromethyl-triflurochloroethyl-ether (see formulae below) but, despite their close relationship, only enflurane can sometimes elicit minor convulsive motions. The same yin–yang kinship exists among barbiturates, which can be turned into convulsants with a chemist's sleight of hand.

Investigators of the mechanism by which drugs produce reversible coma have focused on the cell membrane where lipids and proteins can be affected by substances that alter the wonderful order of these complex structures. Some theorists stress the lipid solubility (think grease stain removers) of anesthetics, others their ability to insinuate themselves in the intricate ways proteins coil up and trap

Table 12.1. GI drugs

Class and agent	Trade name	Dose	Comments
Antacid			
Sodium citrate		p.o.: 15–30 mL	Immediately neutralizes stomach acid
H₂ blockers			i.v. at least 1 h before induction
Cimetidine	Tagamet®	p.o.: 400 mg	More side effects than alternatives
		i.v.: 300 mg	
Famotidine	Pepcid®	p.o./i.v.: 20 mg	
Ranitidine	Zantac®	p.o.: 150 mg	
		i.v.: 50 mg	
Pro-kinetic			
Metoclopramide	Reglan®	p.o./i.v.: 10 mg	Dopamine antagonist to enhance gastric emptying and increase LES pressure

LES: lower esophageal sphincter.

water. Some anesthetics may work by changing the membrane, expanding it, altering its fluidity, and by one or the other or a combination of effects changing cell membrane function and responses to transmitter substances. Many of the organic intravenous drugs, such as propofol, barbiturates, and the benzodiazepines appear to increase the inhibitory action of GABA receptors, while opiates have their Greek alphabet of receptors (see below). From all of this, it must be apparent that we really do not understand all that much about reversibly induced coma or indeed about consciousness itself.

Pharmacologic preparation for anesthesia[1]

Reduce the risk of aspiration (Table 12.1)

The aspiration of acid gastric juice can lead to a nasty chemical burn of the trachea and bronchi and to bronchospasm and pneumonitis and, potentially, to death. We aim to reduce gastric volume and limit acidity. Gastric juice with a pH of 2.5 or less is thought to cause dangerous chemical burns when aspirated. We have several methods to reduce the hazards of aspiration of acidic juice:

(i) Buffer the gastric acid with an antacid. Many different agents are available. We prefer a non-particulate liquid, which not only mixes more readily in the stomach but also causes less harm when aspirated than would be true for a particulate antacid. Sodium citrate (trisodium citrate) or Bicitra® (sodium citrate and citric acid) – which are liquid – find common use in anesthesia. We give 15–30 mL by mouth within 30 minutes before induction of anesthesia.

Table 12.2. Anxiolytics

Agent	Trade name	i.v. dose	Duration	Comments
Diazepam	Valium®	2–10 mg	2–6 hours	Slow i.v.; anticonvulsant, sedative
Lorazepam	Ativan®	1–2 mg	6–8 hours	Sedative
Midazolam	Versed®	0.5–5 mg	2–6 hours	Amnestic
Benzodiazepine Antagonist				
Flumazenil	Romazicon®	0.2–1 mg	60–90 min	Risk of seizures; benzodiazepine withdrawal

(ii) Enhance gastric emptying. Metoclopramide (Reglan®) works both locally – acetylcholine-like and thus enhancing lower esophageal sphincter tone, gastric motility and emptying – and centrally as a dopaminergic blocker. We do not know how much the CNS action contributes to the desired GI effect, but we do know that the drug can cause undesirable CNS effects, including extrapyramidal symptoms; it might contribute to early post-operative delirium. Typical doses for the average adult are 10 to 20 mg by mouth 1 hr (or 10 mg i.v. 30 minutes) before anesthesia.

(iii) Inhibit gastric secretion. We have several drugs that antagonize H_2 receptors and thus inhibit secretion of gastric acid, among them cimetidine (Tagamet®), ranitidine (Zantac®), and famotidine (Pepcid®). We prefer ranitidine (150 mg p.o. or 50 mg i.v.) or famotidine (20 mg p.o. or i.v.) an hour before anesthesia. Proton pump inhibitors (among them omeprazole (Prilosec®), esomeprazole (Nexium®) and pantoprazole (Protonix®)) can also reduce gastric acidity. Because of their slow onset of action (hours), proton pump inhibitors are not routinely prescribed as antacids in anesthesia.

Reduce anxiety (Table 12.2)

Benzodiazepines

To allay fear and induce antegrade amnesia, many patients receive a benzodiazepine before induction of anesthesia. Several different benzodiazepines are on the market. Prominent among them is diazepam (Valium®) and midazolam (Versed®); the latter is about three times as potent as diazepam.

In most adults, small (1–2 mg) intravenous doses of midazolam produce not only a calming effect, but also antegrade amnesia. The effect sets in over 2 to 3 minutes. Benzodiazepines work through GABA receptors, much like alcohol, and therefore, those who are not alcohol-naïve might require additional doses. However, the doses should be separated by at least 2 minutes to avoid missing

Table 12.3. Anti-emetics

Agent	Trade name	i.v. dose	Comments
Droperidol	Inapsine®	0.625 mg	Butyrophenone; dopamine antagonist, anxiolytic
Promethazine	Phenergan®	25 mg	Phenothiazine
Ondansetron	Zofran®	4 mg	Serotonin blocker
Granisetron	Kytril®	1 mg	Serotonin blocker
Dolasetron	Anzemet®	12.5 mg	Serotonin blocker

respiratory depression and even apnea. The elimination half-life is about 3 hours. Midazolam can reduce the incidence of recall of intra-operative events.

Midazolam has also been used to induce anesthesia. We slowly administer 0.2 to 0.3 mg/kg intravenously, and anticipate respiratory depression. Even in small doses, e.g., 1 mg for the average adult, the drug serves as a good anticonvulsant.

As with all CNS active drugs, we use great care in fear of drug interaction, as may occur at the extremes of age or in the debilitated patient.

Flumazenil (Romazicon®) antagonizes the effects of benzodiazepines (see Table 12.2). We titrate it to effect, starting with 0.2 mg given slowly intravenously and not more than a total of 3 mg for the average adult. In case of midazolam-induced respiratory depression, we would manually ventilate the patient's lungs rather than start with an antagonist. Flumazenil can trigger convulsions when given to patients poisoned with tricyclic antidepressants or chronically on high doses of benzodiazepines.

Prevent nausea and vomiting (Table 12.3)

Even though modern anesthesia techniques have decreased the frequency of early postoperative nausea and vomiting, these two disagreeable complications still trouble patients greatly. A number of drugs help to suppress or minimize the occurrence.

Droperidol (Inapsine®)

This butyrophenone is a dopamine antagonist. It has been around for over 30 years and has been used extensively during anesthesia and for the prevention or treatment of nausea and vomiting. We start with 0.625 mg i.v. to the average adult. The question has been raised whether it would be justifiable to give droperidol prophylactically, which would mean giving it to many patients who would not have developed nausea and vomiting. Such across the board prophylaxis can only be defended when the drug poses no risk but offers considerable benefits. Droperidol offers the benefits but not without risks. In 2001, the FDA published a warning implicating droperidol in the prolongation of the QT interval (normal between 0.38 s and 0.42 s, with fast or slow heart rates, respectively). It quoted studies describing patients who developed widening QT intervals exceeding 0.45 s and ending in torsade de pointes, a malignant arrhythmia. Many drugs have been shown to prolong the QT interval, more frequently in women than men. The list includes (but is not limited to) amiodarone (Cordarone®), cisapride (Propulsid®), erythromycin, quinidine, and sotalol (Betapace®). We must be particularly concerned in patients with existing prolongation of the QT interval. We mention the worry about QT prolongation even though in anesthesia a dangerous prolongation of QT intervals had not been linked to droperidol. However, the issue raised by the FDA has caused considerable discussion in anesthesia circles.

Droperidol has other side effects that may be quite troublesome, if not lethal. Very few patients develop extrapyramidal symptoms, others a feeling of terror which they cannot express.

Serotonin receptor blockers

Among these are ondansetron (Zofran®), granisetron (Kytril®), and dolasetron (Anzemet®). These serotonin receptor blockers have found use in patients undergoing chemotherapy and in the prevention of nausea and vomiting postoperatively. The drugs appear more useful as a prophylactic antiemetic rather than in treatment of existing nausea and vomiting. Fortunately, these agents are not burdened with a list of disagreeable side effects (unless you count their cost!) – other than constipation in 11% of patients, something of concern to patients undergoing chemotherapy, and even less frequent headaches and elevated liver enzymes.

Intravenous anesthetics (Table 12.4)

Barbiturates

The drugs with the longest history of intravenous use in anesthesia are the barbiturates. While many different barbiturates have been synthesized and used, the drugs most commonly found in current anesthesia practice are thiopental (Pentothal®) and methohexital (Brevital®). These drugs share the basic barbituric acid foundation (Fig. 12.1), which by itself has no CNS depressant effect. Substitutions on position 5 give us pentobarbital, a slow- and long-acting hypnotic. Simply substituting sulfur for the oxygen on position 2 turns the drug into the highly lipid soluble, fast-acting thiopental.

After an intravenous thiopental bolus, e.g., 4 mg/kg, the patient falls asleep in less than a minute and comes around again within a few more minutes. The drug

Table 12.4. Intravenous anesthetics

Agent	i.v. induction dose	$T_{1/2}$ Elim	Pros	Cons
Etomidate	0.2 to 0.5 mg/kg	2–5 h	Minimal CV depression	Lowers seizure threshold; pain on injection; myoclonus; inhibits steroid synthesis
Ketamine	1 to 2 mg/kg i.m. 5 to 10 mg/kg IM	1–2 h	Maintain ventilation and airway reflexes; excellent analgesia; does not blunt sympathetic nervous system	Dissociative anesthesia → hallucinations; increased salivation; hypertension/tachycardia
Methohexital	1 to 2 mg/kg	4 h	Short half-life oxybarbiturate	Lowers seizure threshold; myoclonus
Propofol	1 to 2.5 mg/kg	0.5–1.5 h	Anti-emetic; short half-life, great for conscious sedation (25 to 75 mcg/kg/min) and TIVA (50–200 mcg/kg/min)	Pain on injection; no analgesia; culture medium for bacteria
Thiopental	2 to 5 mg/kg	12 h	Reliable, inexpensive	Long elimination half-life; histamine release

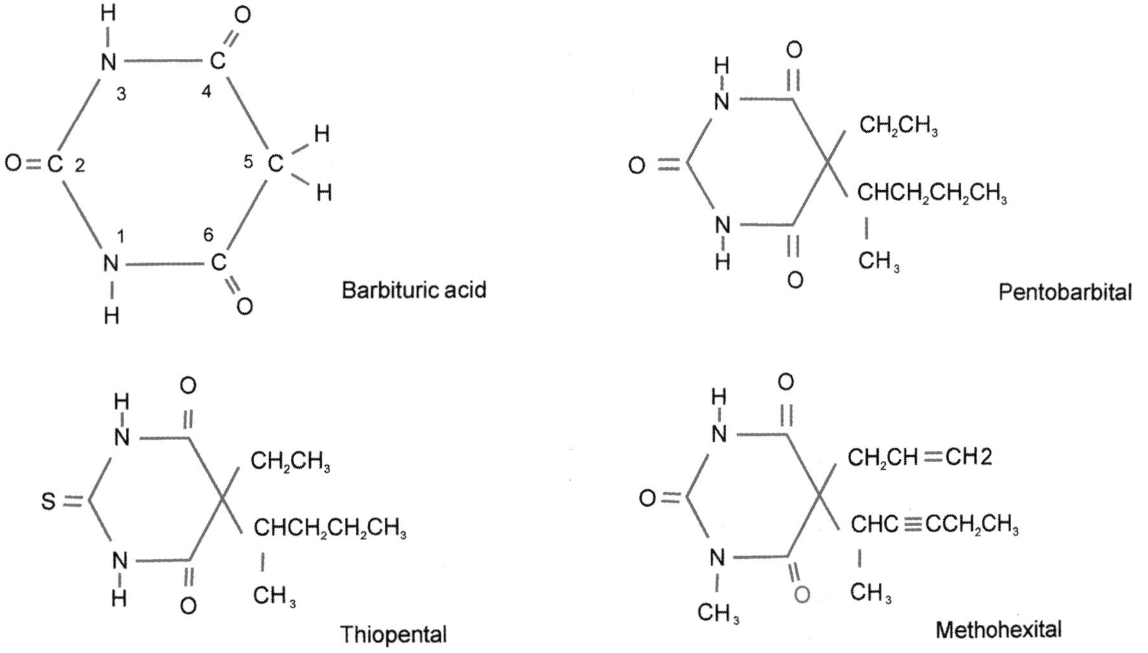

Fig. 12.1 Barbiturate structural relationships. All based on barbituric acid; see the text for a description of the seemingly minor structural variations.

Fig. 12.2 Thiopental distribution. After an intravenous dose of thiopental, the patient's blood levels rise rapidly (not shown here). The blood then distributes the drug according to the hierarchy of blood flow: first to the best perfused vessel rich group (VRG), which includes the brain (also heart, liver, kidneys) where thiopental will exert an early (sleep and cardiovascular effects) and fleeting effect. The other compartments (muscle and fat) then pick up the drug, depending on blood flow and solubility of the drug in the respective tissues. The last compartment, the fat, finally accumulates the drug after the other compartments are already seeing a decline in drug concentration. The fat compartment thus becomes the depot from which the drug trickles back into the blood to be disposed of by biotransformation and excretion.

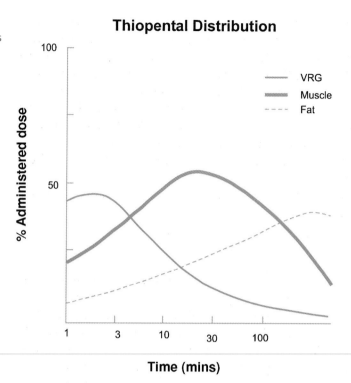

owes its rapid onset of effect to the S= substitution on position 2 and to the fact that the "vessel rich group" (tissues with a high blood flow; especially the brain) gets the first lion's share of the drug. Then the other body compartments pick up more and more drug during the distribution phase, and brain levels fall off rapidly (see Fig. 12.2).

For an animated mental model of this type of drug distribution, see a simulation for a muscle relaxant; the depicted principle applies to other drugs (www.anest.ufl.edu/EA). You will appreciate that much drug not contributing to the primary and desired drug effect lingers in other body compartments. The drug in these "silent" compartments will trickle back into the circulation and the brain for a hang-over effect. Eventually, all of the drug will undergo biotransformation and excretion, but the elimination half-life of thiopental takes about 12 hours. Some of the biotransformation will convert the drug back into an oxybarbiturate (O= instead of S= in position 2), reducing lipid solubility and extending the depressant effect.

Drugs other than thiobarbiturates can have a rapid onset, as exemplified by methohexital, which is a little more potent and more rapidly metabolized than thiopental. All barbiturates used in anesthesia reduce sympathetic control of the peripheral vasculature, thereby increasing the capacitance of the venous system, which in turn leads to reduced preload. Coupled with a negative inotropic effect on the myocardium, blood pressure falls. In compensation, the baroreceptors will accelerate heart rate and mitigate the reduction of cardiac output. Respiration is also depressed. These negative effects do not play a major role in anesthesia of healthy patients where hydration with intravenous fluids can compensate for the reduced preload from venous pooling, and where we routinely overcome depressed ventilation by manual or mechanical ventilation. In addition, the barbiturates tend to constrict the blood vessels in the brain, a welcome side effect when increased intracranial pressure concerns us in patients with tumors or head trauma.

The following non-barbiturates also possess anticonvulsant effects, even in relatively small dosages.

Propofol (Diprivan®)

Propofol is another frequently used intravenous anesthetic. As a phenol, it belongs to an entirely different category of drugs. Not being water soluble, it is presented in a milky-white emulsion of oil, glycerol, and lecithin ("Milk of Amnesia"), an ideal culture medium for bacteria. Sterile technique, of course, is mandatory for all intravenous injections. However, with propofol, we dare not keep an open vial for later use. Because an injection of propofol into a small vein smarts, we often elevate the arm during injection and give it together with a local anesthetic, systemic narcotics, or a tiny dose of thiopental or ketamine. A typical induction dose might be 1 to 2.5 mg/kg. Propofol, 20 to 200 mcg/kg/min, is often given as a continuous infusion for sedation or sleep, for example when a child must hold still for radiation treatment. Together with nitrous oxide (nitrous oxide provides the analgesia, propofol the sleep), it also serves well for short surgical procedures because patients awaken rapidly from this technique and rarely suffer nausea or vomiting.

Propofol also lowers the blood pressure by a negative inotropic myocardial effect, vasodilatation, venous pooling, and reduced preload. It depresses ventilation and reduces cerebral perfusion. Occasionally, patients show mild myoclonic movements during propofol infusion. The drug is cleared from the plasma much more rapidly than thiopental, and the lack of a hangover and freedom from nausea after recovery have secured propofol a place in outpatient anesthesia.

Etomidate (Amidate®)

This drug is chemically unrelated to barbiturates and propofol and enjoys the (perhaps overrated) reputation of causing little cardiovascular depression. It finds use primarily in patients with heart disease where 0.2 to 0.5 mg/kg is given for induction of anesthesia – preferably into a large vein with a rapidly running infusion in order to minimize pain from venous irritation. Etomidate lowers the seizure threshold. In up to half of all patients, it triggers a myoclonus, which appears to be harmless. The drug inhibits cortisol and aldosterone synthesis (via dose-dependent inhibition of 11 β-hydroxylase), a feature that makes it unsuitable for long-term intravenous sedation in the ICU.

Ketamine (Ketalar®)

This drug occupies a peculiar position between the induction agents on the one hand and the narcotic analgesics on the other. It provides both sleep and analgesia – but at a cost. The drug is the grandchild of phencyclidine, a nasty compound that made a brief appearance as an intravenous anesthetic, soon abandoned, and now mainly encountered as a psychedelic drug on the street and known under a medley of colorful names (PCP, Angel Dust, Dust, Sherm, Super Weed, Killer Weed, Elephant, Embalming Fluid, Hog, PCE, Rocket Fuel, TCP). Ketamine has shed almost all of the psychedelic effects of phencyclidine. It provides excellent analgesia (via stimulation of both NMDA[2] and opioid receptors), particularly of the integument and less so of the intestinal tract. It is classified as a dissociative anesthetic because, in low doses, the patient may appear to be awake (perhaps with open eyes and nystagmus) but unresponsive to sensory input. Only in deep anesthesia does the drug obtund airway reflexes, while in light anesthesia with spontaneous ventilation, bronchodilation is a welcome side effect, although increased secretions are bothersome. Unlike the other common anesthetic agents, ketamine *stimulates* the sympathetic nervous system, tending to increase heart rate and blood pressure. As such, it is often the drug of choice in the hypovolemic trauma patient. However, in cardiac patients in congestive failure whose sympathetic system may be exhausted, the drug can reveal its direct myocardial depressant effect. Ketamine would also be relatively contra-indicated for patients at risk of high intracranial pressure, as its sympathetic stimulation increases cerebral blood flow. On awakening from the effect of the drug, many adults, but usually no pediatric patients, experience visual hallucinations and delirium.

In increasing dosages, we use ketamine for analgesia (0.2–0.5 mg/kg i.v.) or for induction of anesthesia (1 to 2 mg/kg i.v. or intramuscularly 5–10 mg/kg). To minimize the frequency of delirium, we give it together with one of the benzodiazepines and to decrease secretions, we add an anti-sialogogue.

Inhalation anesthetics (Table 12.5)

Before discussing the agents one by one, we need to deal with the question of the uptake and distribution of inhaled drugs.

Table 12.5. Characteristics of inhaled anesthetics

Name	Formula	Biotransformed %	Partition coefficients Blood/gas	Fat/blood	Vapor pressure mmHg @ 20 °C	MAC (sea level)
Diethyl ether	$CH_3 - CH_2 - O - CH_2 - CH_3$	20	12	5	440	**1.9**
Enflurane	$H\ FClC - CF_2 - O - CF_2H$	2	1.9	36	172	**1.63**
Methoxyflurane	$CCl_2H - CF_2 - O - CH_3$	50	12	49	23	**0.16**
Halothane	$CF_3 - CHClBr$	20	2.5	51	243	**0.75**
Isoflurane	$CF_3 - CHCl - O - CF_2H$	0.2	1.4	45	238	**1.15**
Desflurane	$CF_3 - CHF - O - CF_2H$	0.02	0.42	27	669	**6.6**
Sevoflurane	$(CF_3)_2\ CH - O - CFH_2$	2	0.6	48	157	**1.8**
Nitrous oxide	N_2O	0	0.47	2.3	38,770	**105**
Xenon	Xe	0	0.12			**56**

The partition coefficients are reported for 37 °C.

Uptake and distribution of inhaled anesthetics

Behind this bland title lurks a concept that has baffled students for years, yet it is fairly straightforward. Here are the facts:

(i) Solubility of the anesthetic in blood has nothing to do with its potency. Indeed, anesthetic effectiveness has to do with the partial pressure of the drug and not with the amount of drug in solution.

(ii) Anesthetics taken up by the blood flowing through the lungs are distributed into different body compartments, depending on the blood flow these compartments receive, the volume of the compartment, and the solubility of the anesthetic agent in that compartment.

(iii) The partial pressure exerted by a vapor in solution has nothing to do with the ambient pressure, but has much to do with the temperature of the solution.

Let us take these three items one by one:

(i) Solubility of the anesthetic in blood has nothing to do with its potency.

Table 12.5 tells the story. At equilibrium, you will find 12 times as much ether (when we say "ether" we refer to diethyl ether; some of the halogenated anesthetics are chemically also ethers, but we call them by their given name, e.g., sevoflurane and desflurane) in blood than in the overlying gas (blood/gas partition coefficient). The blood practically slurps up the ether. Every breath that brings in more ether dumps its load of the anesthetic into the blood perfusing the lungs. It takes breath after breath to deliver enough ether for the blood to come into equilibrium with the alveolar gas. At equilibrium, the partial pressure (but not the concentration per unit of volume) of the ether in the gas phase (alveolar gas) is the same as in the blood.

Fig. 12.3 Conceptual compartments for agent distribution. Drugs are first distributed to the vessel rich group, which receives the majority of the cardiac output. Equilibration here is rapid (both during induction and emergence). The much larger fat compartment receives a much lower blood flow and therefore takes much longer to equilibrate with the agent concentration in blood. While agent in this compartment serves no purpose, resolution of the resulting depot maintains agent in the bloodstream for an extended period of time following discontinuation of the drug administration.

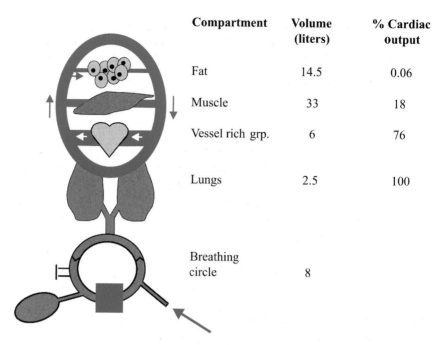

Compartment	Volume (liters)	% Cardiac output
Fat	14.5	0.06
Muscle	33	18
Vessel rich grp.	6	76
Lungs	2.5	100
Breathing circle	8	

We have picked ether (no longer used in the Western world but widely used elsewhere) because of its extraordinary solubility in blood at body temperature. In comparisson, look at sevoflurane. Ether is 20 times as soluble in blood as is sevoflurane. We can quickly bring enough sevoflurane into the alveoli to establish an equilibrium between alveolar gas and blood. For ether, it will take many, many breaths laden with ether to fill the blood compartment and to reach equilibrium between alveolar gas and blood. Yet, diethyl ether and sevoflurane have almost identical MAC values. MAC stands (neither for a computer nor for a truck) for minimal alveolar concentration, namely the concentration in alveolar gas at which 50% of patients no longer respond to a painful stimulus. Thus, when we have attained MAC values for ether and MAC values for sevoflurane, there will be much, much more ether dissolved in the patient than will be true for sevoflurane. It will be quicker to get the patient to sleep – and have him wake up again – with sevoflurane than with ether.

Observe in Table 12.5 that, at equilibrium, you will find five times as much ether in fat than in blood and 45 times as much isoflurane in fat than in blood . . . which brings us to the next point.

(ii) Anesthetics taken up by the lungs are distributed into different body compartments, depending on the blood flow these compartments receive, their volume, and the solubility of the anesthetic agent in that compartment.

Figure 12.3 shows the relationships. Observe the low blood flow and large volume of the fat compartment (not even assuming an obese patient!) and

Table 12.6. Comparison of MAC values for isoflurane at various altitudes

Name of city	Altitude in ft (m)	MAC in % of ambient pressure
La Paz, Bolivia	11 735 ft (3577 m)	1.8%
La Paz, Mexico	33 ft (10 m)	1.15%

the small volume but enormous blood flow to the vessel rich group. These "compartments" are conceptual rather than anatomical; the vessel rich group contains heart and brain as well as kidney and liver.

You can easily imagine that during a long anesthetic, the fat compartment, despite its low perfusion, will accumulate much anesthetic agent because inhalation anesthetics are so very soluble in fat (they make excellent grease stain removers). At the end of the anesthetic, the poorly perfused fat compartment will slowly deliver anesthetic to the venous blood, causing the patient to have a protracted recovery from the anesthetic; the greater the solubility of the agent in fat, the more protracted.

(iii) The partial pressure exerted by a vapor in solution has nothing to do with the ambient pressure, but has much to do with the temperature of the solution.

Water vapor in the lungs at 37 °C has a vapor pressure of 47 mmHg. At that temperature, as many molecules of water leave the blood as enter it. The vapor pressure increases with rising temperatures. At the boiling point, the vapor pressure equals ambient pressure (at the top of the mountain you need to boil your egg a little longer because the water will boil at a lower temperature). At sea level (1 atmosphere or 760 mmHg ambient pressure), it takes 1.15% of isoflurane to render 50% of the population unresponsive to noxious (if the patient were awake the word would be "painful") stimuli. At that barometric pressure, 1.15% equals about 9 mmHg. At altitude with a barometric pressure of 500 mmHg, these same 9 mmHg would be about 1.8% of vapor in the alveolar gas. Thus, the convention of reporting anesthetic concentrations in percent – as our vaporizers do – leaves something to be desired. In Table 12.6, we compare isoflurane MAC values in two cities of very different altitude that happen to have the same name. Remember that about half of our patients will be responsive, i.e., with a movement without being necessarily conscious, at 1 MAC. In order to have almost 100% of patients unresponsive to noxious (painful) stimuli, we need to expose them to 1.3 MAC. Also, remember that most patients have been given other CNS depressants; MAC values change with age (down they go); and distribution of the anesthetic agents also depends on the patient's cardiac output, which, in shock with a very low cardiac output, may send a disproportionate percentage of the blood to brain and heart.

We can anticipate that many CNS depressants will lower MAC. Intuitively not so obvious, however, are reports that hyponatremia, metabolic acidosis, alpha methyldopa, chronic dextroamphetamine usage, levodopa, and alpha-2 agonists can lower MAC, as does pregnancy. We find elevated MAC values in hypernatremia, hyperthermia, and in patients taking monoamine oxidase inhibitors, cocaine and ephedrine. The administration of a sympathomimetic can sometimes lighten anesthesia. Because we always titrate anesthetics to a desired effect and because patients vary greatly in their response to drugs – anesthetics as well as others – these differences in MAC rarely influence our anesthetic practice.

The gases

Only two anesthetic gases (as opposed to vapors) deserve to be mentioned: nitrous oxide and xenon. Cyclopropane and ethylene are two explosive gases used in the past.

Nitrous oxide

Nitrous oxide has been around for centuries and is still widely used. Yet you will often hear it said that, if nitrous oxide were to be introduced today, it would never pass the FDA's muster. For this jaundiced view, we can cite several reasons.

(i) The gas is a weak anesthetic with a MAC of 105%. Thus, it would require a hyperbaric chamber to administer that concentration with enough oxygen to make it safe. In concentrations up to 70% in oxygen, it is an analgesic rather than a reliable anesthetic.

(ii) Because it is such a weak drug, in the past people tended to give high concentrations of it, which is another way of saying that it was given with marginal concentrations of oxygen. Modern anesthesia machines will not let you give less than 25% oxygen, but many patients with ventilation/perfusion abnormalities require a higher FiO_2.

(iii) It does some peculiar things to some important enzymes. By oxidizing vitamin-B12-dependent enzymes (methionine and thymidylate synthetase), it inhibits formation of myelin and thymidine (important in DNA synthesis). Prolonged exposure to nitrous oxide has caused neuropathy and megaloblastic changes as well as leukopenia. A decreased white count was noticed in tetanus patients requiring prolonged mechanical ventilation during which nitrous oxide was used continuously as an analgesic sedative. Attempting to use this effect to advantage, subsequent experiments with nitrous oxide in leukemic patients confirmed the observation that the gas could reduce the white count. Unfortunately, the effect did not last and upon discontinuation of the gas, the cell counts rose back to their pathologic condition. The neuropathic effect of nitrous oxide was observed by a neurologist who saw dentists complaining of different degrees of apraxia, ataxia, and impotence.

Exposure to nitrous oxide was the common denominator in these patients. These effects are not observed during the relatively brief use (minutes or hours instead of repeated use or days of exposure) of nitrous oxide in patients undergoing surgical anesthesia.

(iv) Despite its low blood solubility (blood/gas partition coefficient of 0.47), the high concentration of N_2O administered (50% to 70% in oxygen) causes many liters to dissolve in the body during a lengthy anesthetic. Because it diffuses readily into air-containing bubbles, nitrous oxide can increase the volume of air in the cuff of an endotracheal tube, the gas in the bowel, a bleb in the lung, or gas in the middle ear. The volume of a closed air space, e.g., pneumothorax, will double in just 10 minutes! The doubling time for bowel is *much* slower (hours).

(v) We might also mention that it supports combustion, almost as well as oxygen.

(vi) For neurosurgical procedures, even low-dose and brief exposure to nitrous oxide affects evoked potentials – which we monitor to keep an eye on the integrity of the spinal cord, among other things.

(vii) Based on questionable epidemiologic data and on animal experiments, nitrous oxide has been accused of causing spontaneous abortion in personnel repeatedly exposed to trace concentrations of the gas. Consequently, maximal acceptable trace concentrations of nitrous oxide in the OR have been established by the government: OSHA calls for a time weighted average concentration of less than 25 parts per million.

(viii) Finally, thrill seekers have extensively abused nitrous oxide, obtaining it legally (and stupidly) in the small whippet cylinders. There, the gas exists in its pure form, that is without oxygen. The ill-informed who inhale it from such a source expose themselves to the double trouble of inhaling a hypoxic gas mixture while breathing a harmful gas.

In fairness, we have to say something positive about the gas. Because of its low solubility, it does not take much time to reach equilibrium between alveolar gas and blood, which translates into fairly rapid induction and emergence with minimal cardiovascular side effects. Some pediatric dentists like its mild analgesic effect and the fact that it is tasteless and odorless (which is why industry uses it as a propellant for canned whipped cream). In the pediatric dental practice, nitrous oxide is usually administered in concentrations between 30% and 50% in oxygen. Higher concentrations of nitrous oxide given by itself often lead to excitement. In anesthetic practice, therefore, we administer the gas together with other CNS depressants, for example thiopental or propofol or a halogenated anesthetic vapor.

Even though it has nothing to do with the pharmacology of nitrous oxide, and everything to do with the fact that we give it in high concentrations (up to 70% – whereas the halogenated agents are given in less than 1/10th that concentration), we need to mention three concepts linked to nitrous oxide: the second gas effect; the augmented inflow effect (also called the concentration effect); and diffusion hypoxia.

The second gas effect

If you administer a high concentration of nitrous oxide to the lungs during induction of anesthesia, much of the gas will go into solution in the body, thereby reducing its partial pressure in the lungs. The sum of all partial pressures will equal barometric pressure. In other words, if a large volume of nitrous oxide vanishes, any other (second) (anesthetic) gas present in the lung will experience an increase in its partial pressure, which will speed its uptake by the blood.

The augmented inflow or concentration effect

Because of the large uptake of nitrous oxide, the exhaled volume will be diminished, enabling the next breath to have an increased tidal volume to re-establish normal lung volume.

Diffusion hypoxia

After hours of anesthesia with nitrous oxide, many liters of the gas go into solution in the body. At the end of anesthesia, when the patient no longer inhales nitrous oxide, the liters of nitrous oxide in solution will follow their concentration gradient and be delivered to the lung where the gas will displace other gases – including oxygen. Thus, we give oxygen for a few breaths at the end of anesthesia and thus prevent diffusion hypoxia.

Xenon

This noble gas is even less soluble than nitrous oxide (blood/gas partition coefficient of 0.12) and about twice as potent (MAC = 56%). In addition, it appears to have no major depressant effects on the cardiovascular system. We do not know how it produces anesthesia, being a noble gas (we don't really know how the other not so noble agents do it, either). Xenon would make a desirable anesthetic, were it not for its high cost (about $17/L). Xenon is currently not used in the USA and most studies of the gas come from abroad.

The anesthetic vapors

Ethers

Anesthetic vapors exist as fluids at ambient conditions. They have low vapor pressures, and the vapors overlying the liquid phase have anesthetic properties. It all started with diethyl ether, the granddaddy of anesthetic vapors. Over the last 150 years, uncounted chemists have rearranged the structure of these substances and, by adding halogens, have developed a host of promising anesthetics. Each has distinctive vapor pressures, blood/gas partition coefficients, potencies (see Table 12.5), and side effects, e.g., upper airway irritation, bronchodilation, cardiac irritability.

With the arrival of the non-flammable agents, i.e., halothane (Fluothane®) and the halogenated ethers, we were able to retire from clinical use the highly flammable diethyl ether. Methoxyflurane (Metofane®) was abandoned because of its extensive biotransformation, which led to the liberation of enough fluoride ions to damage the kidneys, causing a vasopressin-resistant high output renal failure. The much less extensive biotransformation of enflurane (Ethrane®) and sevoflurane (Ultane®) also liberates fluoride ions but in such small concentrations that renal problems have not been a cause for concern. Initial worries over nephrotoxicity from sevoflurane's degradation by CO_2 absorbent in the anesthesia circuit (forming the dreaded "Compound A," also known as pentafluorisoprenyl fluoromethyl) appears to lack clinical relevance (unless anesthetizing a rat).

Halogenated aliphatic compounds

So much for the halogenated ethers. Now to a different class, the halogenated aliphatic compounds, the ancestor of which, chloroform ($HCCl_3$), dates back to 1847 when it was first shown to be an anesthetic. While neither irritating nor combustible (a big problem for diethyl ether), it eventually fell out of favor because of its propensity to cause arrhythmias and hepatic damage. A number of other halogenated aliphatic compounds came and went, until finally in the mid 1960s, halothane appeared and was soon widely used. It is still around, even though it had its lumps and bumps. It sensitizes the heart to arrhythmias triggered by catecholamines.

Halothane hepatitis

Soon after the introduction of halothane worrisome reports of "halothane hepatitis" appeared. Fever, malaise, and evidence of liver damage as seen in the elevation of serum aminotransferases pointed to liver damage. Not the halothane molecule itself but the products of its biotransformation cause the trouble. Halothane falls prey to a reductive and an oxidative breakup, the former exaggerated in the presence of hypoxemia, the latter in some patients causing an immune response that can set the stage for severe halothane hepatitis at a future exposure to halothane. Hepatitis after halothane anesthesia is rare (perhaps 1 in 30 000) and much rarer after the other halogenated anesthetics. The extent of biotransformation of the drug might play a role: halothane stands out with 20% to 46% of the agent undergoing biotransformation as compared to isoflurane (0.2% to 2%) and desflurane (0.02%). The products of biotransformation of sevoflurane (2% to 5% metabolized) appear to cause no harm to the liver.

Comparing effects on heart, lung, and brain

All anesthetic vapors affect consciousness and have analgesic effects. They depress ventilation, as judged by decreasing minute ventilation and increasing levels of arterial carbon dioxide, with increasing depth of anesthesia. A few words about generally subtle differences between these drugs:

Inhalation induction

The older halothane and the newer sevoflurane have established for themselves a special niche because they are less irritating to the upper airway than the others. Particularly in children, who abhor needle sticks (and whose veins are more easily cannulated when the child is asleep), anesthesia can be induced quite gently by inhalation of nitrous oxide/oxygen together with either one of these two drugs.

Cardiovascular effects

All volatile agents depress myocardial contractility and cause peripheral vasodilatation. As long as baroreceptors function normally, heart rate will increase in response to hypotension. In deep anesthesia, this compensation will not suffice to prevent a drop in cardiac output. Here, halothane occupies an unusual position. It inhibits the baroreceptor; consequently, we see less tachycardia (even bradycardia in deeply anesthetized children) during halothane-induced hypotension and a greater drop in cardiac output than is true for the other agents at comparable levels of anesthesia. Another oddity regarding halothane anesthesia: otherwise well-tolerated levels of circulating catecholamines, whether injected or liberated by the body, trigger arrhythmias in the presence of halothane.

Respiratory effects

Under very deep anesthesia, ventilation stops, usually before the heart arrests. Thus, a respiratory arrest from an overdose with an inhalation anesthetic need not be fatal if discovered in time, and if ventilation of the (still perfused) lungs with oxygen can remove the volatile anesthetic.

In surgical anesthesia, spontaneous ventilation will still be maintained IF the patient was not given other drugs that depress ventilation – such as opiates – and IF the patient is not paralyzed by neuromuscular blocking drugs, so commonly used in order to relax striated muscles and thus ease the surgeon's job.

In general, all halogenated inhalation anesthetics decrease minute ventilation by decreasing tidal volume. The compensatory increase in respiratory rate cannot prevent a respiratory acidosis (and hypoxemia when breathing room air) because any increase in respiratory rate increases the ventilation of dead space. Respiratory depression and tachypnea are less pronounced with desflurane (Suprane®) and sevoflurane than with halothane, with isoflurane (Forane®) lying somewhere in between.

Table 12.7. Relative potencies of commonly used opioids

	Relative potency	Protein binding (%)	Duration (h)	$T_{1/2}$ (min)
Morphine	1	30	2–3	114
Hydromorphone	8	8	2–3	150
Meperidine	0.1	75	2–4	200
Fentanyl	100	85	1–2	200
Sufentanil	1000	92	0.5	150
Alfentanil	10	90	0.25	85
Remifentanil	200	70	0.1	5

Comparison of the opioids commonly used in anesthesia. $T_{1/2}$ is the time at which one-half of the drug has been eliminated from the body. Clinical duration, however, refers to the approximate duration of drug effect after an intravenous bolus injection. This includes a peak effect (dependent on factors such as lipid solubility (including ionization and pK), volume of distribution, and flow to the effector site) followed by a gradual waning over minutes to hours (redistribution, ion trapping, metabolism). Protein binding significantly affects the volume of distribution, and changes the drug's effectiveness in settings of altered protein binding.

Under inhalation anesthesia, patients respond only sluggishly to rising arterial carbon dioxide levels (= respiratory depression). Even low concentrations of the inhalation agents also depress the chemoreceptor response to hypoxemia.

Central nervous system effects

The inhalation anesthetics depress, in a dose-dependent manner, CNS function – as shown by clinical findings starting with a state of somnolence, during which the patient can still respond – to coma, in which external noxious (we do not call it "painful" as you have to be conscious to find something painful!) stimulation elicits no visible response. This sentence was carefully chosen, because invisible CNS responses are detectable by electroencephalography and evoked potentials; these persist long after motor responses have been abolished. Eventually, they too vanish in deep anesthesia. Halogenated inhalation agents tend to increase cerebral blood flow, which is not a desirable effect in patients at risk of brain swelling. In neurosurgical anesthesia, we rely greatly on intravenous techniques using the inhalation agents only in low doses and as adjuncts.

The opioids (Table 12.7)

Today, narcotics play a major role in general anesthesia. Their advantage lies in their potent ability to abolish pain without depressing the heart. Their principle

Fig. 12.4 Carbon dioxide response: effect of opioids. Rising carbon dioxide blood levels cause ventilation to increase. In very high concentrations, carbon dioxide becomes a depressant and even anesthetic. Opiates typically shift the carbon dioxide response curve to the right and flatten it. The degree of shift depends on the drug and the dose. Very high doses stop ventilation all together, as seen all too often in "dead on arrival" victims of heroin overdose. In anesthesia, we sometimes give narcotics to the point of causing apnea (and intense analgesia) – while maintaining normal $PaCO_2$ levels by providing mechanical ventilation.

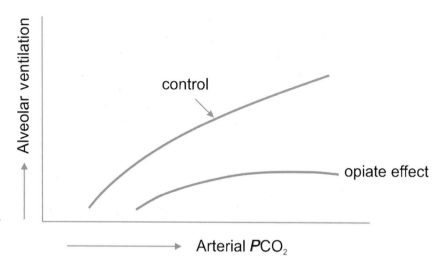

side effect remains powerful respiratory depression resulting in a decreased respiratory rate and finally respiratory arrest (Fig. 12.4). This side effect can be tolerated if we are prepared to ventilate the patient's lungs, as we do routinely when patients receive neuromuscular blocking drugs and thus require mechanical ventilation. Unchecked respiratory depression and elevation of arterial carbon dioxide can reduce resistance in the arterial bed of the cerebral circulation, leading to increased intracranial pressure. Chemoreceptor depression by opioids reduces the respiratory response to hypoxemia; however, the administration of oxygen to a hypoxemic patient may further depress ventilation, demonstrating that chemoreceptor activity still contributes to the respiratory drive.

At this time in anesthesia, we have no useful opioid that would spare the μ-2 receptors responsible for respiratory depression, while exerting a full effect on the receptors apparently involved in analgesia (μ-1, δ-1, δ-2 and κ-3 for supraspinal analgesia, and μ-2, δ-2 and κ-1 for spinal analgesia). As mentioned in the brief historical piece, to be eaten alive by a lion may not be painful, presumably because the endogenous opioid polypeptides (the enkephalins, endorphins, dynorphins and neoendorphins) kick in – evidently without causing fatal respiratory depression but presumably allowing for a gasp. We tend not to rely on this physiologic response to gourmand lions, even with the most fearsome of surgeons at work.

Opioids exhibit many side effects other than respiratory depression. Interesting to anesthesia are the depressant effects on the autonomic nervous system with a decrease in sympathetic tone and a preponderance of vagal activity, leading to bradycardia and a reduction in blood pressure. The observed hypotension after large doses of opioids gives evidence of venous pooling (exaggerated in patients with a reduced blood volume) rather than a direct depressant effect on the heart. Meperidine, having vagolytic effects, behaves somewhat differently.

During a cholecystectomy, we need to be aware that opioids can increase the tone of the sphincter of Oddi, thereby increasing pressure in the biliary system and interfering with a surgeon's attempt to perform a cholangiogram.

Opioids have numerous side effects in addition to respiratory depression. These range from miosis (the infamous pin-point pupils – again meperidine is the exception), itching, constipation and nausea, to changes in mood (either euphoria or dysphoria, depending on the setting and the patient). Some of these effects have their origin locally (constipation), others centrally (chemoreceptor stimulation triggering nausea).

By now the opioids have amassed quite a retinue of narcotic compounds, some of which appear to have unrelated chemical footprints. While heroin, codeine, and many relatives show their kinship with morphine, others are classified as piperidines and phenylpiperidines, comprising meperidine and the different fentanyl drugs.

Morphine

Morphine (Fig. 12.5) has a long tradition as an analgesic for wound pain with a typical i.m. dose of 10 mg for a 70 kg patient. Despite its propensity to stimulate histamine release, we make extensive use of i.v. morphine for management of acute pain, as an intra-operative analgesic and adjunct to general anesthesia, and post-operatively as the most common drug for patient-controlled analgesia (PCA). We also commonly administer morphine neuraxially (epidural or subarachnoid) to obtain 18–24 hours of post-surgical analgesia, though delayed respiratory depression remains a concern. One of its metabolites, morphine-6-glucuronide, retains much of morphine's activity and has been implicated in prolonged respiratory depression observed in patients with renal failure.

Meperidine (pethidine, Demerol®, Dolantin®, Pethadol®)

Another synthetic opioid, meperidine, deserves to be mentioned, though in anesthesia we use it less today than before the arrival of its chemical grandchildren, the fentanyls. Meperidine (Fig. 12.5), with 1/10 the potency and shorter duration of action than morphine, occupies a unique spot among opioids in its antimuscarinic activity. Patients receiving meperidine do not develop the "pin-point pupils" we expect with other opioids; they may also become tachycardic and complain of a dry mouth. The drug can be associated with nausea and vomiting as well. Most importantly, it should not be given to patients taking monoamine oxidase inhibitors because severe respiratory depression, excitation, and even convulsions can be the consequence (serotonin syndrome). Meperidine's main metabolite, normeperidine, lasts for days ($T_{1/2}$ elimination $= 15$–40 h). Particularly in the setting of impaired renal function, the accumulation of normeperidine can cause myoclonus and seizures.

Fig. 12.5 Opioid structures.

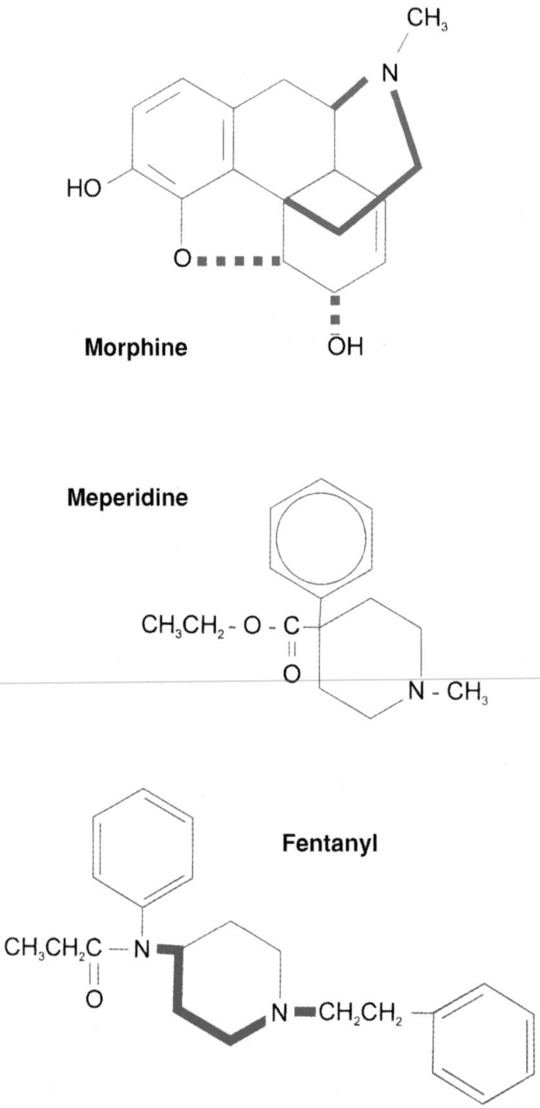

Morphine

Meperidine

Fentanyl

Fentanyls

Fentanyl (Sublimaze®) (Fig. 12.5), with a potency 100 times that of morphine, has even more potent offspring. The growing list includes 3-methyl fentanyl, lofentanyl, and etorphin being several thousand-fold as potent as morphine. None have made it into the operating room. Nor are they needed as potency in the clinical setting means relatively little as long as the desired effect can be reached by adjusting the dose, and as long as that dose can be readily delivered. Clinical

Table 12.8. Opioid antagonist

Agent	Trade name	i.v. dose	Comments
Naloxone	Narcan®	0.1–0.4 mg	Duration 1–2 hours; may elicit withdrawal syndrome in addicts; reverses analgesia as well

doses of the fentanyls are all in the microgram/kg range, thus posing no difficulty to intravenous administration.

The differences among the fentanyls reside primarily in the duration of action, since, in general, the respiratory depressant effect runs parallel with the analgesic effectiveness. There are small differences in the onset of action after an intravenous bolus, with fentanyl and sufentanil (Sufenta®) taking about 6 minutes for the peak effect to set in while alfentanil (Alfenta®) and remifentanil (Ultiva®) reach their peaks in about a minute. Remifentanil, an ester, deserves special mention as the only narcotic that falls prey to non-specific plasma esterases that hydrolyze the drug, thus rapidly curtailing its effect. The other opioids have to rely on liver blood flow and hepatic biotransformation. A comparison of each of the commonly used opioids may be of help (Table 12.7).

Finally, let us mention that narcotic addiction has not spared anesthesia and nursing personnel. Easy access to narcotics has been blamed for the higher frequency of addiction among anesthesia personnel than other health care workers.

Opioid receptor antagonism: naloxone (Narcan®)

Opioids are antagonized by naloxone, chemically related to morphine and competing for receptor sites occupied by the agonists (See Table 12.8). In the adult, we usually start with 40–100 mcg naloxone intravenously, expecting to see a response within a minute. The half-life of the drug is around 40 minutes. Thus, patients who had been depressed by the longer acting drugs, such as morphine, must be observed for at least an hour in order not to miss recurring respiratory depression. In addicted patients under the influence of and tolerant to large doses of a narcotic analgesic, a larger dose of naloxone can trigger a stormy withdrawal reaction, as can administration of some of the mixed agonist-antagonist drugs, among them butorphanol (Stadol®) and nalbuphine (Nubain®). These latter agents have a ceiling effect on respiratory depression, a property considered vital in obstetrics where they are commonly used – never mind that the patient's pain is not much relieved by these agents!

Table 12.9. Analgesics for moderate to severe pain (VAS 5 to 7) in adults

Generic name	Equivalent dose	Duration	Dose	Found in trade name products
Codeine	100 mg p.o.	3–4 hours	0.5–1.0 mg/kg q4 h max 60 mg/dose	60 mg codeine with acetaminophen in Tylenol #3®
Fentanyl	50 mcg i.v.	1–2 hours	0.5 mcg/kg i.v. PCA: 0.3 mcg/kg with 6 min lockout	Sublimaze®. Also available as Duragesic® transdermal patch
Hydrocodone	15 mg p.o.	3–4 hours	5–15 mg p.o. q4–6 h	2.5–7.5 mg hydrocodone with acetaminophen in Vicodin® & Lortab®
Hydromorphone	0.75 mg i.v. 3.75 mg p.o.	2 hours	2–4 mg p.o. q4–6 h 0.5–2 mg i.v. PCA: 0.005 mg/kg with 6 min lockout	Dilaudid®
Meperidine Pethidine	150 mg p.o.	1–3 hours	50–150 mg p.o. q3–4 h 25 mg i.v. PCA: 10 mg with 15 min lockout	Demerol®, Pethadol®
Morphine sulfate immediate release	5 mg i.v. 15 mg p.o.	2–4 hours	10–30 mg p.o. q4 h 0.04 mg/kg i.v. PCA: 0.02 mg/kg with 6 min lockout	Roxanol®
Oxycodone immediate release	10 mg p.o.	3–4 hours	0.05–0.15 mg/kg p.o.	Roxicodone® 5 mg oxycodone with acetaminophen in Percocet®, Roxicet® & Tylox® 4 mg oxycodone with aspirin in Percodan®
Tramadol[a]	100 mg p.o.	4 hours	50–100 mg q4–6 h max 400 mg/day	Ultram®
	2 tablets p.o.	4 hours	2 tabs q4–6 h max 8 tabs/day	37.5 mg tramadol with acetaminophen in Ultracet®

[a] Tramadol is a centrally acting, non-opioid analgesic, though it has some activity at μ receptors. Unlikely to be equianalgesic with the opioids.

Table 12.10. Analgesics for mild pain (VAS < 5) in adults

Generic name	Trade name	Dose	Duration
Acetaminophen	Tylenol®	650–1000 mg q4–6 h max 4000 mg/day	4 hours
Ibuprofen	Motrin®; Advil®	200–800 mg q6–8 h max 3200 mg/day	6 hours
Ketorolac	Toradol®	20 mg load then 10 mg q4–6 h max 40 mg/day for 5 days	4 hours
Naproxen	Naprosyn®	250–500 mg BID	8 hours
Naproxen sodium	Alleve®	550 mg BID	

Clinical perspectives on the use of analgesics

In the chapter on Post-operative care, you will find a discussion of how to assess the severity of pain. Many different drugs find use in the treatment of pain. The following tables are not intended to guide therapy, but are presented here for the sake of orientation. We do not offer a discussion of these drugs and urge the reader to consult pharmacologic texts and the information offered by the manufacturers. For moderate to severe pain (VAS 5 to 7), you may see one of the drugs in Table 12.9 prescribed. For mild pain we often use one of the common oral, non-narcotic analgesics that are available over the counter (Table 12.10).

Neuromuscular blockers and their antagonists (Table 12.11)

Even though the title presents the official name, we will call them muscle relaxants with the understanding that we are talking about drugs used in anesthesia to facilitate tracheal intubation and to ease the surgeon's work. The good news about muscle relaxants is that they affect only striated, voluntary muscles, but not the myocardium and the smooth muscles under autonomic control (including the uterus). Being quaternary ammonium compounds, all muscle relaxants carry a charge and thus do not readily cross the blood–brain barrier (no effect on the brain) or the placenta (no effect on the fetus). The bad news is that the relaxants do not spare the muscles of ventilation. That fact has cost many lives when partially paralyzed patients became hypoxemic because inadequate ventilation was allowed to persist during and particularly after anesthesia. Do not forget that muscle relaxants have no anesthetic effect, that a patient paralyzed by muscle relaxants has no way of signaling that he is in pain, uncomfortable or short of breath, a fact not lost on those patients suffering intra-operative awareness. There

Table 12.11. Non-depolarizing muscle relaxants by duration of action

Generic name and class	Trade name	Intubating dose[a]	Biotransformation/ excretion	Comments
Benzylisoquinolines				
Short acting:				
Mivacurium	Mivacron®	0.2 mg/kg	Plasma pseudocholinesterase	Histamine release
Intermediate acting:				
Atracurium	Tracrium®	0.4 mg/kg	Hoffman elimination and esterases	Histamine release
Cisatracurium	Nimbex®	0.2 mg/kg	Hoffman elimination and esterases	
Long acting:				
Doxacurium	Nuromax®	0.06 mg/kg	Renal (80%)	
Steroid nucleus				
Short acting:				
None at present				
Intermediate acting:				
Vecuronium	Norcuron®	0.2 mg/kg	Hepatic (80%)	
Rocuronium	Zemuron®	0.8 mg/kg	Hepatic (70%)	
Long acting:				
Pancuronium	Pavulon®	0.1 mg/kg	Renal (80%)	Tachycardia
Pipecuronium	Arduan®	0.085 mg/kg	Renal (60%)	

[a]A higher dose is often used for rapid sequence induction.

are far too many reports of recall of intra-operative and ICU events when muscle relaxants were employed. Note also that even the pharmacological reversal of the effect of muscle relaxants has undesirable side effects. Whenever muscle relaxants are used, we assume great responsibility for the safety of the patient. Many procedures do not require muscle relaxants. When no muscle relaxants are used, the patient can breathe spontaneously, which they tend to do very well indeed as long as we are not heavy handed with CNS depressants. Muscle relaxants are usually divided into depolarizing and non-depolarizing drugs.

Depolarizing muscle relaxants

Succinylcholine (Anectine®) is the only depolarizing drug still in use. It has been around for 50 years and has served us well because of two characteristics: it is rapid in onset and short in duration, being hydrolyzed by plasma cholinesterases.

Indeed, perhaps as much as 90% of the intravenously injected drug is hydrolyzed before reaching the effector site at the neuromuscular junction. Patients deficient in plasma cholinesterase will be paralyzed for several hours from a standard intubating dose of 1 mg/kg, which should last for only 5 minutes or so.

Cholinesterase deficiency can be genetic or acquired. One in 3200 patients (less often in Oriental and African peoples) may be homozygous for atypical cholinesterase. When we suspect this because of a family history or a previous anesthetic complication, we can test the patient's plasma in vitro, using dibucaine (Nupercaine®), a local anesthetic. Dibucaine strongly (80%) inhibits normal or 'typical' plasma cholinesterase but not the atypical cholinesterase (20%). A report of a 'dibucaine number' of 80 is good news, suggesting that the patient is homozygous for typical plasma cholinesterase. A dibucaine number of 20 or so would be found in a patient homozygous for atypical plasma cholinesterase, who would have an abnormally protracted effect from succinylcholine. Dibucaine numbers between these extremes suggest a heterozygous genetic make-up. In the patient heterozygous for normal plasma cholinesterase, the succinylcholine effect is likely to be doubled or tripled (5 to 15 minutes). Incidentally, patients homozygous for atypical cholinesterase are quite asymptomatic – as long as no one gives them succinylcholine or other drugs dependent on hydrolysis by plasma cholinesterases. We see the acquired deficiency – characterized by decreased blood levels of normal plasma cholinesterase – in patients exposed to organophosphates (chemical warfare and pesticides) and those on echothiophate (for glaucoma) who would also more slowly break down some other esters such as local anesthetics of the ester type.

Succinylcholine does not compete with acetylcholine at the neuromuscular junction; instead, it depolarizes the muscle and in so doing, it opens ion channels, much like acetylcholine does, but the channels stay open much longer. Potassium begins to leak out and serum potassium levels can rise by 0.5 mEq/L after an intubating dose (succinylcholine 1 mg/kg). In damaged (crush or burn injuries) or degenerating muscles (after spinal cord injury or in muscular dystrophy), this potassium leakage can be exaggerated to the point where the cardiac effects of hyperkalemia become life-threatening. The risk of yet unrecognized muscular dystrophy, together with the potential for a bradycardic response, has limited the use of succinylcholine in children. Succinylcholine has several additional undesirable properties. Before paralysis sets in, it causes fasciculation of striated muscle, a feature that has been blamed for post-operative myalgia experienced by some patients and for a transient rise in intragastric and intracranial pressures. By a mechanism not well understood, intra-ocular pressure also rises briefly after an intubating dose. Therefore, we do not use the drug in patients with an open eye lest the patient lose vitreous. In the past, succinylcholine was often used as a continuous infusion. In that application, it loses its advantage of a short-acting depolarizing blocker because the patient will develop a so-called phase II block that looks as if the patient had been given a non-depolarizing muscle relaxant (see chapter on Monitoring).

When tracheal intubation fails and the succinylcholine effect wears off, we might be tempted to administer a second dose of succinylcholine within a few minutes of the first dose. This is dangerous, possibly causing severe bradycardia and even asystole presumably triggered by cholinergic effects of the second dose. Therefore, always administer i.v. atropine or glycopyrrolate (0.6 mg or 0.4 mg, respectively, for the average adult) before giving a second dose of succinylcholine.

Non-depolarizing muscle relaxants

The South American Indians did not know that they were delivering a non-depolarizing drug in their blowpipes when hunting monkeys. We might wonder if they were astonished that they were not weakened or paralyzed when eating the curare-poisoned monkey meat. Being quaternary, bulky molecules, D-tubocurare is not absorbed from the gut. Today, we have a long list of non-depolarizing muscle relaxants, which act by competing with acetylcholine at the neuromuscular endplate. They are either benzylisoquinolines (like the original D-tubocurare) or steroid derivatives. We can roughly classify them as short-acting, i.e., less than 30 minutes, intermediate-acting (between 30 and 60 minutes), and long-acting (over 1 hour). The duration is affected by the dose and by how we define duration. For example, an intubating dose (a lot of relaxation!) of a short-acting drug might provide adequate surgical relaxation (soft abdominal muscles) for $1/2$ hour; however, after these 30 minutes, the patient might not be capable of maintaining normal blood gases without assisted ventilation. Table 12.10 provides a short list of some of the currently used drugs with certain of their characteristics. For each drug we give an "intubating dose."

In Fig. 12.6 we show mivacurium (Mivacron®) representing the benzylisoquinolines and pancuronium (Pavulon®) for its steroid nucleus. Observe the ester linkage in mivacurium, which can be attacked by cholinesterases, making it a short-acting drug; however, subject to prolonged effect with plasma cholinesterase deficiencies.

Muscle relaxant reversal

We do not reverse the effect of succinylcholine with an antagonist. Instead, we unwearingly ventilate the patient's lungs until the block has worn off, even if that takes hours in a patient homozygous for atypical cholinesterase. This differs from the non-depolarizing drugs. An excess of acetylcholine, the physiologic transmitter substance at the endplate, will compete with the non-depolarizing relaxant for access to the endplate. Thus we give a cholinesterase inhibitor, prolonging the life of acetylcholine so it can better compete. Because these inhibitors act not only

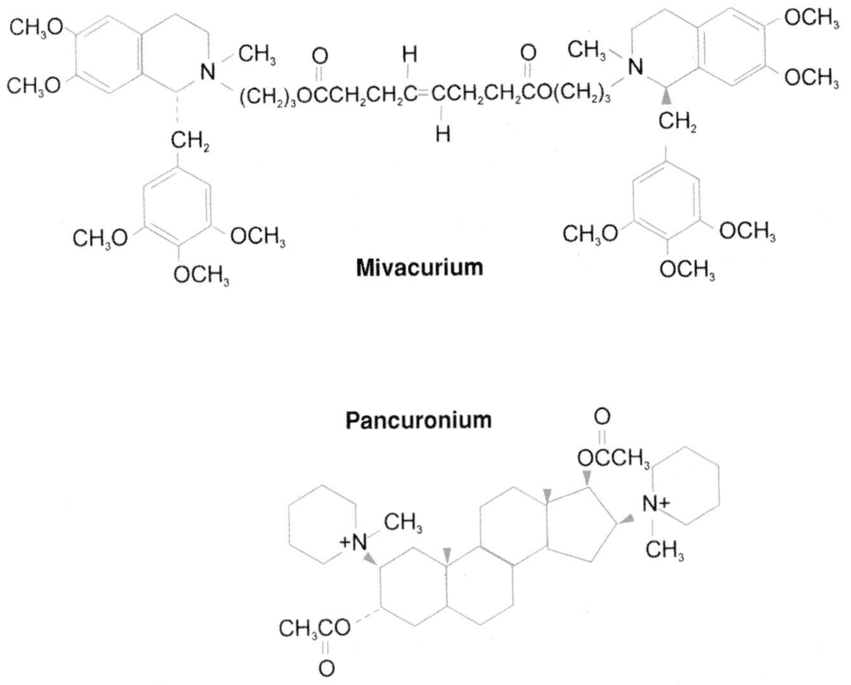

Fig. 12.6 Neuromuscular blocking agent structures.

on the neuromuscular apparatus but also generate an excess of acetylcholine at autonomic sites, we add an anticholinergic drug that acts primarily on the autonomic (muscarinic) receptors. Thus, atropine or glycopyrrolate (Robinul®) can prevent the unwanted autonomic effects of the cholinesterase inhibitors, such as excessive salivation, bradycardia and intestinal cramping.

The most commonly used cholinesterase inhibitors are neostigmine (Prostigmin®) and edrophonium (Tensilon®). Both are quaternary ammonium compounds that do not cross the blood–brain barrier, and both are potent cholinesterase inhibitors. While they show small differences in their action, either one can serve when the weakening effect of a muscle relaxant must be reversed. Neostigmine takes up to 10 minutes after an intravenous dose to reach its peak effect; edrophonium is much faster. Reversal of neuromuscular blockade cannot be achieved unless a few receptors are unblocked to give acetylcholine a fighting chance. Using a "twitch monitor" (see Monitoring), we do not administer reversal agents until we detect at least a small response to stimulation (indicating that no more than 90% of the receptors are blocked). Typical reversal doses are:

neostigmine up to 0.08 mg/kg or edrophonium up to 1 mg/kg

with

atropine or glycopyrrolate up to 15 mcg/kg.

These doses must be adjusted to meet the patient's requirements (see Table 12.12).

Table 12.12. Antagonists to neuromuscular blocking agents

Agent	Trade name	i.v. dose	Comments
Cholinesterase inhibitors; administer with atropine or glycopyrrolate to prevent bradycardia			
Edrophonium	Tensilon®	1 mg/kg	Duration 10 min
Neostigmine	Prostigmin®	0.08 mg/kg	Duration 60 min
Pyridostigmine	Mestinon®, Regonol®	0.2 mg/kg	Duration 90 min
Physostigmine	Antilirium®	1 mg	Duration 60 min; crosses blood–brain barrier; counteracts central cholinergic syndrome

A new category of drugs, the cyclodextrins, now in clinical trials, might offer advantages. They appear to chelate the muscle relaxants without antagonizing them via the inhibition of cholinesterases.

The Monitoring chapter details assessment of neuromuscular blockade and muscle strength.

Dantrolene

Dantrolene (Dantrium®) finds use as an oral medication in the treatment of muscle spasms in multiple sclerosis, cerebral palsy, stroke, or injury to the spine. It affects skeletal muscles directly, i.e., beyond the neuromuscular junction. In the treatment of malignant hyperthermia, we count on its ability to re-establish a normal level of the dangerously elevated ionized calcium in the myoplasm. We start with a bolus of 1–2 mg/kg, repeated every 5–10 minutes as necessary, to a maximum of 10 mg/kg. The drug comes in vials containing 20 mg dantrolene and 3000 mg mannitol. This has to be dissolved with 60 ml sterile water. To administer 2–3 mg/kg to an adult will require many vials and an extra pair of hands to prepare and administer the drug.

The local anesthetics (Table 12.13)

Instead of flooding the whole system, from head to toe, with an inhalation or intravenous anesthetic, we can inject an anesthetic locally; directly on a nerve; place it into the epidural or subarachnoid space, catching several nerves at once; or paint or spray it on mucous membrane as a topical anesthetic. Local anesthetics come in two chemical classes: esters and amides, with tetracaine (Pontocaine®)

Table 12.13. Local anesthetics

Agent	Trade name	Relative potency	Duration	Maximum dose for infiltration
Esters				
Chloroprocaine	Nesacaine®	4	Short	800 mg
Procaine	Novocain®	1	Short	1000 mg
Tetracaine	Pontocaine®	16	Long	100 mg
Amides				
Bupivacaine	Marcaine®	4	Long	175 mg
Etidocaine	Duranest®	4	Long	300 mg
Lidocaine/ lignocaine	Xylocaine®	1	Short + epi: Moderate	Plain: 300 mg (4.5 mg/kg) + epi: 500 mg (7 mg/kg)
Mepivacaine	Polocaine®, Carbocaine®	1	Moderate	400 mg
Ropivacaine	Naropin®	3	Long	300 mg

Lidocaine

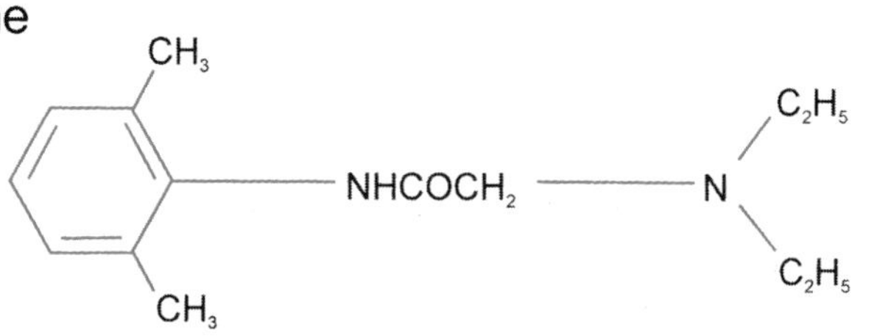

Tetracaine

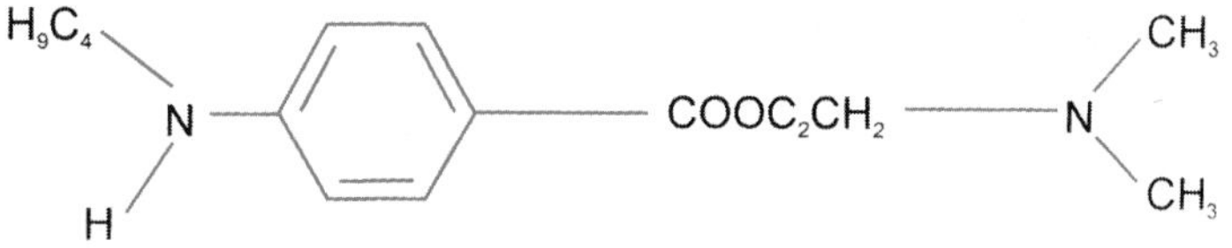

Fig. 12.7 Local anesthetic structures.

being a well-known ester and lidocaine (Xylocaine®) an even better known amide (Fig. 12.7). A trick for remembering the class of local anesthetics: if there is an 'I' before the "caine" it is an amIde. The trick to the trick, though, is this only works for the *generic* name of the drug, e.g., bupivacaine is an amide, even when found in a bottle labeled Marcaine®.

Local anesthetics interfere with nerve conduction by blocking ion fluxes through sodium channels. This blockade occurs from the inside of the cell. Local agents are weak bases with pKb (pH at which half of the base is ionized) values between 8 and 9; at a lower pH, more of the drug will be ionized and vice versa. Only the lipid-soluble, non-ionized form can penetrate cell membranes. Once inside, the cationic form of the drug is favored because the interior of the cell tends to be more acidic than the outside. This is fortuitous, since the cationic form will go to work on the ion channel. In general, an acidic medium – for example, inflamed tissue – will favor ionization and thus delay penetration of the drug, while an alkaline medium (such as adding bicarbonate to a highly acidic commercial preparation of lidocaine) can hasten the movement of the drug through membranes.

Different nerves exhibit different sensitivities to local anesthetics. We see the clinical evidence of this during spinal anesthesia where the block for cold sensation and sympathetic activity extends to higher dermatome levels than for other sensations and motor activity. This is commonly attributed to resistance to blockade provided by the thick, heavy myelin sheath coating the motor (Aα) fibers, which is lacking on the skinny non-myelinated preganglionic sympathetic (B) fibers and postganglionic sympathetic and dorsal root (C) fibers. However, the picture is quite complex. The sensitivity will also be influenced by the position of the nerve in a nerve bundle exposed to the local anesthetic, the speed of nerve conduction, and by how much of the nerve must be exposed to the anesthetic to block it.

Once injected or applied to a membrane, the drug will be carried away by the blood. To delay this, we often add epinephrine to the local anesthetic, which constricts blood vessels, thus decreasing tissue perfusion and prolonging the local anesthetic effect. It does not take much epinephrine. Solutions of as little as 1 to 800 000 have been found to do the trick. However, frequently we add epinephrine (adrenaline) in a concentration of 1 to 200 000 so that if we inject into the blood stream (rather than around the nerve), the patient will get a little tachycardia, alerting us to stop the injection immediately. Greater epinephrine concentrations will not further prolong the local anesthetic effect, but will cause more tachycardia (experienced by patients as "butterflies in the stomach," headache, and apprehension). The drugs are metabolized according to their structure: the esters fall prey to plasma cholinesterase and undergo hydrolysis. Microsomal enzymes in the liver go to work on the amides. Occasionally, the products of biotransformation of local anesthetics cause mischief, for example some patients are allergic to *para*-aminobenzoic acid, which forms during ester hydrolysis. Methemoglobinemia (and reduced oxygen carrying capacity) has been observed after the use of prilocaine (Citanest®) and benzocaine, the latter a topical anesthetic (with a sad history of causing contact dermatitis) found in some sprays.

Lidocaine has seen widespread use as an antiarrhythmic drug. Its mechanism of action as a local anesthetic also works on the heart muscle where it can block sodium channels. This can explain its effect on phase IV depolarization, and thus decreased excitability and automaticity. The therapeutic effect of small intravenous doses of lidocaine (1 mg/kg as a bolus or 40 mcg/kg/min as an infusion – up or down titrated to effect) alert us to the fact that local anesthetics do have cardiac effects, not all of which are welcomed. Dangerous cardiac toxicity (hypotension, A–V block, ventricular fibrillation) has been triggered by bupivacaine mistakenly injected intravenously. All local anesthetics can have such cardiac toxicity; however, it is a particular problem with bupivacaine as its duration of binding with sodium receptors is much longer than that of other agents. Importantly, victims of bupivacaine-induced cardiac toxicity have survived after *prolonged* resuscitation.

Local anesthetics will also affect the central nervous system when injected intravenously or when a large peripheral dose is rapidly absorbed. Thus, both procaine and lidocaine have been used as intravenous anesthetics. However, their margin of safety is too narrow to recommend their routine use. With overdose, convulsions are common. As many as 4 out of 1000 patients might exhibit some CNS excitation during a regional local anesthetic. Typically, the patients complain of numbness around mouth and tongue, dizziness, tingling, and tinnitus, and they often become restless before seizing. We treat seizures with manual ventilation with oxygen and a small intravenous dose of, for example, thiopental (20 to 50 mg bolus for the average adult) or midazolam (1 mg bolus).

We have a large selection of local anesthetics available. The drugs differ primarily in their duration of action. Depending on dose and concentration, we have at our disposal everything from the long-acting tetracaine (Pontocaine®), bupivacaine (Marcaine®) and etidocaine (Duranest®), to the short-acting chloroprocaine (Citanest®) and procaine (Novocain®). Lidocaine and mepivacaine fit into the intermediate category.

Additives

Bicarbonate
As mentioned above, we add bicarbonate to those drugs prepared at a particularly acidic pH (lidocaine, chloroprocaine) to speed onset of anesthesia (it also reduces burning when making a skin wheal).

Epinephrine
We might add epinephrine to the local anesthetic solution to (i) prolong the duration of anesthesia, particularly for vasodilating local anesthetics such as lidocaine; (ii) reduce peak plasma concentration of the local anesthetic, also more important for vasodilating agents; (iii) increase the density of regional anesthetic

blocks (by an unknown mechanism); and (iv) as a marker for intravascular injection. Because of epinephrine instability in an alkaline environment, commercial local anesthetic preparations containing epinephrine are highly acidic. We can add bicarbonate, and/or use plain local anesthetics to which we add epinephrine ourselves. Remember that 1:200 000 epinephrine is only 5 mcg/mL – use a tuberculin syringe and measure carefully! Important note: because we fear necrosis of the tip we do not add epinephrine to blocks placed at an "end organ," e.g., digits, penis, nose, ears.

Clonidine (Catapres®)

Through unclear mechanisms, small doses of clonidine enhance and prolong regional anesthesia. One mcg/kg added to the local anesthetic for a Bier block appears to delay the onset of tourniquet pain. In epidural and spinal anesthesia, 50 to 75 mcg clonidine has been found to augment the effect of both local anesthetics and opioids.

Opioids

We add opioids to neuraxial anesthetics to prolong the analgesic effect. Manageable side effects include itching, nausea, and vomiting. Respiratory depression, though less common, concerns us greatly, and we usually employ pulse oximetry on the post-surgical ward. Neuraxial morphine carries a risk of delayed respiratory depression, so we continue to monitor about 24 hours after the last dose.

Bronchodilators

Bronchospasm, a common problem, whether related to asthma or chronic obstructive lung disease, can be treated with bronchodilators. These include primarily phosphodiesterase inhibitors and beta-adrenergic drugs.

Two phosphodiesterase inhibitors, aminophylline (Phyllocontin®; Truphylline®) and theophylline (Theo-Dur® and many others), cousins to caffeine, can be infused intravenously. Patients not previously exposed to the drugs receive a loading dose and then a continuous infusion aiming for serum concentrations associated with bronchodilation. Serum levels in excess of 25 mcg/mL are associated with seizures and arrhythmias.

Among the β_2-adrenergic bronchodilators, albuterol (Ventolin® and many others) and terbutaline (Brethaire®) find common use for inhalation. Albuterol has a longer duration of action (up to 6 hours) than terbutaline (up to 3 hours). Even though they are beta$_2$ agonists, some patients develop beta$_1$ effects, such as tachycardia and arrhythmias. Therefore, caution should be exercised in administering them to cardiac patients in whom tachycardia would be dangerous.

Cardiovascular drugs

The anticholinergic drugs

While numerous anticholinergic drugs exist, in anesthesia we deal almost exclusively with atropine and glycopyrrolate, and occasionally with scopolamine. All three drugs act on the autonomic nervous system, blocking the effect of acetylcholine at post-ganglionic nerve endings. Thus, they accelerate heart rate (if sympathetic tone is present and capable of accelerating heart rate), bronchodilate, cause mydriasis (thereby increasing intraocular pressure), inhibit salivation (and in the process dry secretions in the upper airway), inhibit sweating (by blocking the effect of postganglionic sympathetic cholinergic stimulation), and exert a variety of effects on the GI and GU systems. In anesthesia we use atropine or glycopyrrolate to counteract bradycardia, salivation, and intestinal cramping, all of which are side effects of neostigmine.

Atropine and scopolamine are tertiary amines and thus capable of crossing the blood–brain barrier. In the elderly, scopolamine often causes delirium. Both drugs cross the placenta, and atropine has been observed to accelerate fetal heart rate. Both drugs have a dual effect – in addition to their well-recognized peripheral anticholinergic effect, they have a stimulating central vagal effect. With scopolamine, we sometimes see bradycardia when the central stimulating effect outlasts the peripheral blocking effect of the drug. Glycopyrrolate is a quaternary, charged compound and thus largely prevented from crossing the blood–brain barrier or the placenta.

Drugs to raise blood pressure (Table 12.14)

Hypotension is initially treated with intravenous fluids, lightening of anesthesia, and asking the surgeon not to compress major vessels such as the vena cava (if that was responsible for reducing preload). Sometimes elevating the legs and thereby increasing venous return can help to improve cardiac output and arterial blood pressure. In addition, several drugs are available to improve myocardial contractility, increase arterial resistance, and decrease venous capacitance through adrenergic effects (Table 12.14).

Ephedrine

The old standby still finds common use. We rely on its three-armed effects, alpha and beta stimulation as well as a release of norepinephrine from postganglionic sympathetic nerve terminals. Ten to 20 mg intravenously will increase heart rate and arterial pressure and stimulate the CNS, which we usually do not observe when we give the drug during anesthesia. It has a duration of action of about 20 minutes.

Table 12.14. Drugs to raise blood pressure

Drug	Receptors	Effects	Infusion mixture	Infusion rate	Notes
Amrinone		↑contractility ↓SVR	500 mg in 500 mL = 1 mg/mL	5–10 mcg/ kg/min	First must bolus with 0.5–2.0 mg/kg; phosphodiesterase inhibitor; may cause thrombocytopenia
Calcium chloride		↑contractility			Slow bolus 1–10 mg/kg; direct action on myocardium; arrhythmogenic, particularly with hypokalemia
Digoxin		↑contractility ↓HR in SVT			Slow bolus 0.125–0.25 mg; delayed onset and low therapeutic safety ratio
Dobutamine	β_1	↑HR (slight) ↑contractility	500 mg/250 mL = 2 mg/mL	1–20 mcg/ kg/min	Greater increase in contractility than HR, despite β_1 mechanism
Dopamine	α_1 β_1	↑HR (slight) ↑contractility bronchodilation ↑SVR (high dose)	400 mg/500 mL = 800 mcg/mL	1–20 mcg/ kg/min	Direct and indirect; <10 mcg/kg/min β_1 >10 mcg/kg/min $\alpha_1 > \beta_1$
Ephedrine	α_1 β_1 β_2	↑HR ↑contractility bronchodilation			Mixed direct and indirect; duration 10–60 min; preserves uterine blood flow
Epinephrine	α_1 α_2 β_1 β_2	↑HR ↑contractility bronchodilation ↓SVR (low dose) ↑SVR (high dose)	1 mg/250 mL = 4 mcg/ mL or 4 mg/250 mL = 16 mcg/mL	0.05–0.15 mcg/ kg/min	Arrhythmogenic; 1–2 mcg/min: β_2 4–10 mcg/min: β_1 10–20 mcg/min: $\alpha_1 > \beta$; diverts flow from kidneys to skeletal muscle; produces uterine vasoconstriction
Isoproterenol	β_1 β_2	↑HR ↑contractility bronchodilation ↓SVR	4 mg/250 mL = 16 mcg/mL	0.025–0.15 mcg/ kg/min	i.v. duration 1–5 min; arrhythmogenic
Norepinephrine	α_1 α_2 β_1	↑↑ SVR ↓CO	4 mg/250 mL = 16 mcg/mL	0.05–0.15 mcg/ kg/min	Massive ↑ SVR → HTN and reflex ↓HR
Phenylephrine	α_1	↑↑SVR	40 mg/250mL = 160 mcg/mL	1–3 mcg/kg/min	Reflex ↓ HR; no vasoconstriction of CNS vessels
Vasopressin		↑↑SVR	100 u/100 mL = 1 u/mL	0.2–0.9 u/min	Bolus dose 40 u; vasopressor during cardiac resuscitation and refractory hypotension

Mix all catecholamines in D_5W to prevent oxidation. HR = heart rate; SVR = systemic vascular resistance; CO = cardiac output; HTN = hypertension; SVT = supraventricular tachycardia.

Epinephrine/norepinephrine

Epinephrine (adrenalin in Britain) and norepinephrine (and noradrenalin) are the two catecholamines we find circulating in blood. Norepinephrine is liberated from sympathetic nerve terminals and the adrenal medulla, while epinephrine comes only from the adrenal gland. Chemically, these two transmitter substances are identical but for a methyl group on the amine gracing epinephrine but not *nor*epinephrine (NOR = N Ohne (German for "without") Radical). The drugs do what sympathetic stimulation does. Being physiologic transmitter substances, these catecholamines have a fleeting effect. Single bolus injections last only for a matter of a few minutes.

The body makes extensive use of these catecholamines when fight, fright, or flight call for cardiovascular, pulmonary, muscular, ocular, and intestinal adjustments. It is amazing how well these substances with overlapping adrenergic effects orchestrate their actions to an optimal end-result of sympathetic stimulation. Clinically, we are limited to giving one drug or the other, counting on just one or the other effect. For example, low doses of epinephrine may reduce blood pressure a little through a beta$_2$ effect, while larger doses raise pressure and accelerate heart rate. With norepinephrine, we see primarily increased pressure without tachycardia – as long as the baroreceptors are active. Typical doses used in the operating room might start with 10 to 20 mcg of epinephrine as a single i.v. bolus to help the average adult patient through a spell of hypotension, for example during anaphylaxis. Usually reserved for more dire situations, we titrate a norepinephrine infusion to effect, starting perhaps with 0.1 mcg/kg/min. Epinephrine can also be given by continuous infusion. During cardiac resuscitation when we assume the body to have become very much less responsive to circulating catecholamines, doses as high as 1 mg epinephrine as a bolus have been used.

Dopamine

A biochemical forerunner to norepinephrine, dopamine also finds clinical use. It has the – undeserved – aura that in low rates of infusion, e.g., 1–3 mcg/kg/min, it can support blood pressure while maintaining renal perfusion and promoting diuresis. In larger concentrations, it turns into a vasopressor with renal vasoconstriction, just as norepinephrine, which it can liberate from post-ganglionic sympathetic terminals.

Dobutamine (Dobutrex®)

A synthetic catecholamine, dobutamine is a selective β_1 agonist with greater effect on contractility than heart rate. It improves cardiac output in patients in cardiac failure. Because of its rapid metabolism, we administer dobutamine as an infusion at 2 to 10 mcg/kg/min, titrated to effect.

Table 12.15. Drugs to lower blood pressure

Drug	Mechanism of action	Onset	Duration	Adult i.v. dosage	Comments
Esmolol	β_1 blockade $\rightarrow$ $\downarrow$CO	1–2 min	10–20 min	0.25–1.0 mg/kg bolus	
Labetalol	α_1 β_1 β_2 blockade $\rightarrow$ $\downarrow$SVR and $\downarrow$CO	1–5 min	2–4 h	10–25 mg divided doses	
Nitroglycerin	Direct venodilator	1 min	10 min	0.5–10 mcg/kg/min	Drug of choice in myocardial ischemia
Nitroprusside	Direct arterial and venodilator	0.5 min	2–4 min	0.2–8 mcg/kg/min	Disrupts cerebral autoregulation; causes cyanide toxicity in high doses
Hydralazine	Direct arterial dilator	10–20 min	3–4 h	5–10 mg bolus	Often used in pre-eclampsia
Verapamil	Direct arterial and venodilator; $\downarrow$contractility	1–2 min	5–15 min	0.05–0.2 mg/kg over 2 min	Prolongs conduction time

CO = cardiac output; SVR = systemic vascular resistance.

Isoproterenol (Isuprel®)

Another synthetic catecholamine, isoproterenol activates both β_1 and β_2 receptors with great vigor (2–10 times the potency of epinephrine). We use this agent to (i) increase heart rate, (ii) decrease pulmonary vascular resistance, and (iii) rarely, bronchodilate (i.v. or as an aerosol). Typical of β_1 agonism, heart rate, contractility and cardiac output increase while β_2 vasodilation reduces SVR. The net effect is a fall in diastolic and mean blood pressures. Isoproterenol also induces arrhythmias.

Phenylephrine (Neosynephrine®)

An old standby, phenylephrine sees vasoconstrictive service in nose drops and as an intravenous, pure α_1 agonist. We expect to see both venous and arterial vasoconstriction with the typical intravenous bolus of 40 to 100 mcg, which should raise blood pressure for about 5 minutes. Because of its relatively short duration of effect, we can also infuse it at a rate of about 10 to 100 mcg/min (titrated to effect). Lacking effects at the β receptors, the drug will not increase heart rate or contractile force. Instead, a baroreceptor response can lead to lower heart rates.

Drugs to lower blood pressure (Table 12.15)

While deepening the anesthetic or adding opioids will correct hypertension from light anesthesia, many patients require further blood pressure control. We have many agents at our disposal, with varying mechanisms of action.

Beta blockers

The older propranolol (Inderal®) was not selective and blocked both β_1 and β_2 receptors, thus getting some patients into trouble with bronchoconstriction. Nevertheless, when it became available it represented a major advance in the treatment of hypertension, myocardial ischemia, and ventricular arrhythmias.

Frequently used today are labetalol (Normodyne®; Trandate®) and esmolol (Brevibloc®), two beta-blockers selective for the β_1 receptors with just a weak β_2 blocking component. Labetalol has the added advantage of some α_1 blocking effect, perhaps 1/7th as strong as its β_1 effect, thus enhancing its antihypertensive action with a little peripheral vasodilatation. It has a long duration of action, lasting several hours. Typical intravenous doses start with 10 mg for the average adult. If necessary, these doses can be repeated in 2- or 3-minute intervals, three or four times.

Esmolol has two characteristics that make it useful in special circumstances: it exerts a prominent effect on heart rate and has a rapid onset and relatively short duration with a half-life of under 10 minutes. The typical bolus dose is 0.25–1.0 mg/kg while infusions of 50 mcg/kg/min may be used for a more sustained effect.

Beta blockers are widely used in anesthesia where the common tachycardia secondary to surgical stimulation or with tracheal intubation can lead to a mismatch of myocardial oxygen supply (reduced time for coronary perfusion) and demand (tachycardia, particularly when matched with hypertension). In addition to its intra-operative use, several studies have demonstrated that prophylactic use of beta blockers, e.g., metoprolol, throughout the perioperative period reduces cardiac morbidity and mortality. This is particularly true for patients with coronary artery disease.

When an elevated blood pressure cannot, or should not, be lowered by beta blockade or by deepening anesthesia, and particularly when we wish to have minute-to-minute control of blood pressure, we need agents with rapid onset of action and short duration. To meet this need routinely, the body liberates nitric oxide from the vascular endothelium, which has a fleeting effect of relaxing vascular smooth muscle. Two frequently used drugs, nitroglycerin and nitroprusside, appear to work by forming nitric oxide, so intimately involved in the tone of blood vessels. Both drugs take effect within a minute and will dissipate within 5 minutes. A direct vasodilating hypotensive agent, hydralazine (Apresoline®), finds less use because of its slow onset (up to 10 minutes) and its long duration (up to 4 hours) of action. However, its long, safe track record makes it a favorite in the obstetric suite.

Nitroglycerin

Widely used in cardiology in the treatment of angina, nitroglycerin dilates vascular smooth muscle, with a preponderance of effect on venous over arterial vessels. For angina, a typical dose might be a 0.4 mg tablet under the tongue. As a hypotensive agent to lessen intraoperative bleeding, we infuse nitroglycerin intravenously at a rate of 0.5 to 1 mcg/kg/min. It is important to permit such low doses time to show their effect before adjusting the dose upward (potentially up to 10 mcg/kg/min in tolerant patients) in order to avoid hypotension and a stormy up and down of blood pressure by impatiently adjusting the infusion rate.

Nitroglycerin has the reputation of relieving coronary spasm and subendocardial ischemia, and thus it finds use when ST-segment depression or flipped T waves signal myocardial distress. Reduced ventricular pressure and cardiac output, without a marked rise in heart rate, help to re-establish a favorable balance of myocardial oxygen demand and supply.

Sodium nitroprusside (Nipride®)

In doses similar to those for nitroglycerin, i.e., starting an infusion of 0.5 to 2 mcg/kg/min and up to 10 mcg/kg/min, if needed, nitroprusside appears to have a more pronounced effect on arterial vessels and the pulmonary vascular bed than nitroglycerin. In the brain, sodium nitroprusside dilates vessels and interferes with autoregulation, which can present problems to patients at risk of increased intracranial pressure. The biotransformation of nitroprusside can lead to methemoglobinemia and, in extreme cases, to the liberation of cyanide. To minimize the chance of this toxicity, we monitor the total dose and keep it well below 0.5 mg/kg/h.

Clonidine (Catapres®)

Clonidine occupies an interesting position in the classical scheme of drugs. On the one hand, it looks a little like a catecholamine, without chemically belonging to this category; on the other hand, it stimulates alpha adrenergic receptors – but α_2 instead of α_1. Thus, it inhibits adrenergic stimulation and decreases sympathetic influence on the heart and peripheral vascular bed, resulting in bradycardia and hypotension. As such, the drug finds use in the treatment of hypertension. Anesthesiologists must be aware that the sudden discontinuation of clonidine medication can trigger rebound hypertension.

Clonidine also produces mild sedation and analgesia. It has been used both orally and mixed with local anesthetics to enhance and prolong analgesia (see Local anesthetic additives).

Nitric oxide

This interesting gas hides behind a mouthful term, namely the "endothelium-derived relaxing (vasodilatory) factor" or EDRF for short. Its precursors reside in neurons, vascular endothelium, and macrophages. Once synthesized intracellularly, the very short-lived nitric oxide (NO) triggers a cascade of steps leading to the relaxation of vascular smooth muscle. As soon as a potential therapeutic role of NO had been appreciated – without a full understanding of its different physiologic roles – industry made it available as a gas that now finds application in treatment

Table 12.16. Antiarrhythmic drugs[a]

Agent	Trade name	i.v. dose	Comments
Adenosine	Adenocard®	6–12 mg	To convert PSVT to sinus rhythm, if only briefly; may cause bronchospasm; Duration <10 s; administer rapidly
Amiodarone	Cordarone®	300 mg	For atrial and ventricular arrhythmias; high doses linked to pulmonary toxicity
Atropine		0.6–1.0 mg	Anticholinergic; treats bradycardia
Diltiazem	Cardizem®	20 mg	Calcium channel blocker; starting dose for conversion of PSVT, or control of ventricular rate in patients with atrial fibrillation or flutter
Epinephrine		1 mg	For cardiac arrest; high dose epinephrine no longer recommended
Glycopyrrolate	Robinul®	0.4 mg	Anticholinergic; quaternary amine that does not cross the blood–brain or placental barriers
Lidocaine	Xylocaine®	1 mg/kg bolus or 30 mcg/kg/min	For stable ventricular tachycardia and ventricular arrhythmias
Procainamide	Procan®, Pronestyl®	20 mg/min	Alternative for lidocaine-resistant arrhythmias
Verapamil	Calan®, Isoptin®	2.5–10 mg	Calcium channel blocker to treat PSVT; may increase conduction in accessory pathways

PSVT: paroxysmal supraventricular tachycardia.

[a]Beta-blockers: Agents with activity at β_1 receptors would be included in this group, see above under Drugs to lower blood pressure

of patients with acute respiratory distress syndrome (ARDS). Short-term inhalation of tiny concentrations of NO (about 20 ppm) appears to be beneficial in this difficult clinical syndrome.

Antiarrhythmic drugs (Table 12.16)

Peri-operatively, we see more tachycardias (light anesthesia) than bradycardias (which might be an ominous sign of profound hypoxemia or in children an indication of all too deep anesthesia), and we treat them according to their etiologies. That is, we would not give beta blockers to reduce heart rate if light anesthesia must be held responsible for the rapid rate, nor would we give atropine to treat hypoxemia-induced bradycardia.

For the treatment of arrhythmias of the atria and ventricles, we have a large selection of fairly specific drugs from which we have picked a few that find frequent use in anesthesia and/or cardiac life support (Table 12.16). Both atropine and glycopyrrolate can be used to treat symptomatic bradycardia. However, in patients with acute myocardial ischemia, raising the heart rate can be dangerous because it will increase oxygen demand.

Table 12.17. Drugs used in advanced cardiac life support

Agent	i.v. dose	Comments
Bicarbonate	0.5 to 1 mEq/kg	Treat acidosis and hyperkalemia
Vasopressin	40 units	Vasopressor during cardiac resuscitation and perhaps refractory hypotension

Adenosine as a drug occupies a special niche because the body itself synthesizes this fleeting byproduct of ATP. We use it primarily in the treatment of re-entrant AV node tachycardias such as paroxysmal supraventricular tachycardia (PSVT). Even if the rhythm fails to convert to sinus, the transient slowing of the tachycardia can help with a specific diagnosis.

Lidocaine and procainamide work not only as local anesthetics (lidocaine better than procainamide) but also as useful antiarrhythmic drugs in the treatment of ventricular extrasystoles. Two calcium channel blockers deserve mention: diltiazem and verapamil. Both find use in the treatment of a variety of supraventricular arrhythmias and by slowing AV conduction, they can reduce heart rate in patients in atrial fibrillation.

Advanced cardiac life support

Many drugs already discussed also appear in manuals on cardiac life support, for example in the treatment of arrhythmias and hypotension. The two drugs presented in Table 12.17 not yet mentioned deserve a brief note. In the past, sodium bicarbonate was given in cardiac arrest probably more often than useful. Currently, the American Heart Association recommends it for the treatment of pre-existing hyperkalemia, in diabetic ketoacidosis, in patients overdosed with tricyclic antidepressants or cocaine, and to alkalinize the urine in aspirin poisoning. We usually start with 1 mEq/kg and then, if possible, check arterial blood gases before giving more. Vasopressin, a relatively new addition to the list of drugs used in advanced cardiac life support, powerfully constricts vessels. A single dose of 40 units has been used instead of epinephrine in patients in ventricular fibrillation who had failed to respond to three shocks.

NOTES

1. Throughout the text we use generic names for drugs. Most drugs have several trade names of which we give at least one commonly used in the USA.
2. *N*-methyl-D-aspartate.

Part III

Clinical cases

In the following eight cases, we briefly describe anesthetic approaches, issues, and some potential complications. The reader will find many of the points discussed in the first two sections of the book applied in the management of these cases. An alternative is a problem-oriented approach, namely first to read the cases and then, primed with many questions, delve into the first two sections of the book.

Clinical talk teems with acronyms. Some abbreviations used throughout the cases include:

ABG: arterial blood gas.
ABP: arterial blood pressure (from an invasive arterial catheter).
ACE: angiotensin-converting enzyme.
ACT: activated clotting time.
Airway: read the Airway evaluation chapter to understand the examination.
aPTT: activated partial thromboplastin time.
ASA: American Society of Anesthesiology physical status classification.
BIS: bispectral index.
BP: blood pressure.
BUN: blood urea nitrogen.
CPAP: continuous positive airway pressure.
CPP: cerebral perfusion pressure.
Cr: creatinine.
CV: cardiovascular system.
ETT: endotracheal tube.
fb: finger-breadth (the width of an average adult's finger).
Hct: hematocrit.
HR: heart rate.
ICP: intracranial pressure.
NPO: *nil per os* = nothing by mouth.
NSR: normal sinus rhythm.
PAC: pulmonary artery catheter.
PACU: post-anesthesia care unit.
PCWP: pulmonary capillary wedge pressure.
Plt: platelet count.
PT: prothrombin time.
S1, S2, S3, S4: the first through fourth heart sounds, respectively
SpO_2: oxyhemoglobin saturation by pulse oximetry.

Breast biopsy under conscious sedation

The following case will emphasize conscious sedation and its potential complications.

Learning objectives:

- general pre-operative evaluation
- sedative agents
- respiratory depression: detection, management
- mask ventilation
- laryngeal mask airway
- reversal of sedation.

The patient, a 40-year-old and otherwise healthy woman, comes for breast biopsy.

This procedure is usually performed in two stages: first a radiologist places a needle percutaneously into the lump. Next, the patient reports to the operating room for removal of the lump, pathologic confirmation of the margins, and perhaps a larger procedure depending on the circumstances.

History: She has no chronic medical problems but recently detected a lump in her right breast. Needle localization was performed in radiology this morning and she now presents to the operating suite for lumpectomy.

This healthy patient requires very little additional anesthetic work-up. We ask about the following:

(i) a brief review of systems, including gastro-esophageal reflux disease (*negative*)

(ii) past surgical procedures (*none*)

(iii) family history of anesthetic problems (*none*)

(iv) current medications, including over-the-counter herbal remedies (*none*)

(v) allergies, including latex (*none*)

(vi) habits including smoking, alcohol and drugs (*none*)

(vii) physical examination, including airway:

Nervous white woman in no acute distress; weight 60 kg; height 5′4″ (165 cm)
BP 120/80 mmHg; HR 80 beats/min; respiratory rate 12 breaths/min

Airway: Mallampati I, 4 fingerbreadth(fb) mouth opening, 4 fb thyromental distance, full neck extension
CV: S1, S2 no murmur
Respiratory: Lungs clear to auscultation
Dressing with needle in right breast.

(viii) pre-operative laboratories and studies *(none are indicated)*
This healthy patient would be classified as ASA 1.

Anesthetic preparation: We discuss the risks/benefits of the various anesthetic options. She selects i.v. sedation and we administer an anxiolytic (midazolam (Versed®) 2 mg i.v.).

The surgeon will inject a local anesthetic, blunting the majority of the pain from the procedure, while the anesthesiologist is present to observe and reassure the patient, administer additional anxiolytics or opioids, and treat any hemodynamic instability. Most patients prefer not to be awake and aware during such a procedure. Anesthetic options include (i) conscious sedation, in which the patient remains arousable and in control of her own airway, but free from anxiety and generally unaware of the procedure, and (ii) general anesthesia in which the airway must be managed by mask, laryngeal mask airway or endotracheal tube. After we explain the risks to the patient, she selects i.v. sedation.

Establishment of sedation: Once in the operating room, we apply standard monitors (non-invasive blood pressure, ECG, pulse oximetry), taking care to avoid the right arm for blood pressure cuff application in case axillary node dissection becomes necessary. Following a 50 mg bolus of propofol, we start an infusion at 50–80 mcg/kg/min. The patient's saturation declines to 95% so oxygen via nasal cannula is applied at 4 L/min and the saturation rapidly returns to 100%.

In order to obtain a therapeutic blood level rapidly, we give an initial bolus of propofol and follow it with a continuous infusion to maintain the level of sedation. When the patient is sufficiently drowsy, positioning, prepping and draping can commence. While it should not be necessary, everyone in the room must be reminded the patient is "awake." This includes a sign on the door for those entering later. Unfortunately, the decorum of the OR is not routinely suitable for the awake patient. As in any workplace, discussions may depart from the task at hand, causing concern for a patient who is aware, and might recall irrelevant or objectionable talk.

Maintenance of anesthesia: We titrate the propofol infusion to the desired effect with a goal of arousability with slurred speech, but respiratory and hemodynamic stability.

During injection of local anesthetic into the breast, she complains of pain. We administer fentanyl 50 mcg, and increase the propofol infusion rate. One minute later the patient moans and we respond with another 50 mcg fentanyl. Fifteen minutes later the SpO_2 is falling rapidly. On examination we discover she is apneic. We start ventilation by mask, but encounter difficulty maintaining an open upper airway. When things do not get much better after placing an oral airway, we insert a laryngeal mask airway (LMA) and achieve good air movement. Her saturation rebounds rapidly.

Less than 2 mcg/kg fentanyl should not cause apnea. Alone, that is usually true, however opioids combined with sedatives act synergistically to depress ventilation. Had we been monitoring respiratory pattern/rate we would have noticed that her breathing became dangerously slow a couple of minutes after we had given fentanyl. Our detection method (pulse oximetry here) failed us because we gave so much supplemental oxygen that her PaO_2 was probably close to 200 mmHg as long as she was breathing, if slowly. Thus she had to be almost apneic for her PaO_2 to fall below 80 mmHg, where a drop in the SpO_2 would be expected.

In this case a smaller dose of fentanyl might have been more appropriate, or perhaps the use of a shorter acting opioid such as remifentanil. More importantly, we should monitor respiratory rate, either via a precordial stethoscope (impractical for this particular surgical procedure) or by a capnograph attached through the nasal cannula. At the first sign of oversedation, we could have breathed for her and administered a reversal agent (naloxone). However the side effects of reversal must also be considered, particularly in the middle of an operation.

In managing the apnea, several issues need be recognized. If the problem is central, e.g., oversedation impairing respiratory drive, the patient's lungs will have to be manually ventilated. If soft tissue obstruction of the upper airway is to blame, we need to establish an open airway with the help of an oral airway or LMA. In this difficult phase of being neither awake nor completely anesthetized, manipulation of the upper airway can lead to laryngospasm, coughing, vomiting, and significant movement (usually much to the dismay of the surgeon). In our case the problem was central depression and the patient tolerated the LMA. At this point we usually add nitrous oxide and increase the propofol infusion rate so she will continue to tolerate the device. This increased sedation is limited by the need to have her resume spontaneous ventilation.

Emergence from anesthesia: During closure of the incision, we titrate down the propofol and eventually discontinue the nitrous oxide. When the bandage has been applied, and the patient is awake and breathing with a good respiratory pattern, we suction the posterior pharynx and remove the LMA.

Post-anesthesia care. There should be little pain from this procedure. We turn the care of the patient over to the postanesthesia care unit (PACU) nurses with standing orders of morphine for pain, and an anti-emetic, as needed.

One advantage of the LMA is that, if the patient is breathing spontaneously but not fully awake, she can be transported to the PACU with the LMA in place, where the nurse removes it at the appropriate time.

Discharge: When the patient is fully awake and tolerating oral intake, she can be discharged home with a caregiver, prescription for an analgesic and instructions not to drive for 24 hours.

Carpal tunnel release under Bier block

The following case will describe the use of intravenous regional anesthesia.
  Learning objectives:
- pre-operative management of the asthmatic patient
- intravenous regional anesthesia
- local anesthetic toxicity
- intra-operative bronchospasm.

A 50-year-old asthmatic woman comes for carpal tunnel release.

This minor procedure is usually performed as an outpatient. That is, the patient comes in the day of surgery, and returns home afterward.

History. She has frequent painful tingling of her right hand, consistent with carpal tunnel syndrome. Her past medical history is significant only for asthma since childhood. The asthma is controlled with albuterol metered dose inhaler (MDI) three times a day and more if necessary. She has never had surgery, and gives no family history of anesthetic complications. She takes only asthma medications and hormone replacement therapy. She has no allergies, but smokes two packs a day with a 50 pack-year smoking history. She drinks socially and takes no illegal drugs.

We will ask this patient additional questions regarding her lung disease, to determine its severity, as well as whether her current medical therapy is optimal.

The patient describes chronic asthma without identified precipitating factors or seasonal variation. She has never been intubated for an asthmatic attack, but has been to the emergency room on several occasions. The last event was more than 2 years ago. She has not received steroids but has required extra doses of her MDI twice in the last week, which is about normal for her. She has not had a cold in the last 2 weeks. She has no recent pulmonary function tests (PFTs) or chest radiographs.

Pulmonary function tests are unlikely to alter our anesthetic management for this peripheral operation. Her medical therapy appears to be adequate.

Physical examination: Caucasian woman in no acute distress; weight 85 kg; height 5′ 4″ (160 cm)
BP 135/80 mmHg; HR 90 beats/min; respiratory rate 16 breaths/min

Airway: Mallampati I, 4 fb mouth opening, 4 fb thyromental distance, full neck extension
CV: S1, S2 no murmur
Resp: Lungs with mild bilateral expiratory wheezes; mildly lengthened expiratory phase; no obvious use of accessory respiratory muscles.

While we require no pre-operative laboratory or other studies in this ASA II patient, bedside peak flow testing may be useful.

Asthmatic patients are at increased risk for intra-operative bronchospasm and post-operative pulmonary complications. Avoiding instrumentation of the airway reduces this risk, therefore we prefer local or regional anesthesia.

Anesthetic preparation: We discuss risks/benefits of local anesthesia/intravenous sedation vs. intravenous regional anesthesia (IVRA) vs. regional anesthesia vs. general anesthesia; the patient selects IVRA. We administer nebulized albuterol followed by an anxiolytic (Midazolam (Versed®) 2 mg i.v.)

We will perform an IVRA.

Establishment of regional anesthesia. Once in the operating room, we apply standard monitors (without using the right arm), including nasal cannula with a CO_2 sensor. We place a second i.v. in her right hand, and then apply a double tourniquet to the upper arm. We squeeze out all blood currently in the arm by holding it up and tightly wrapping it in an elastic bandage. Then we inflate the tourniquet to about 100 mmHg above her systolic pressure. After injecting 50 mL of 0.5% plain lidocaine (in divided doses with a test aspiration every 10 mL) into the i.v. below the tourniquet (not the other i.v.!), we remove the catheter. Her arm will appear blanched and she will have a pins and needles sensation, then no sensation at all. We titrate sedation using propofol at 50–80 mcg/kg/min. This sedative is a particularly good choice in the asthmatic patient.

Everyone in the room should be aware the patient is awake.

Maintenance of anesthesia: We titrate the propofol infusion to effect, maintaining arousability to speech and an acceptable respiratory rate. Suddenly the patient complains of ringing in her ears and tingling around her mouth.

These are common early signs of local anesthetic toxicity. We check the tourniquet to insure the pressure is adequate, and perfusion of the arm has not returned. We ask the surgeons about bleeding at the surgical site and monitor the patient closely for sequelae of local anesthetic toxicity including seizures and cardiovascular collapse.

We immediately inflate the second tourniquet cuff and the symptoms subside. After 30 minutes the patient complains of pain at the site of the tourniquet. She is becoming restless and the surgeons still need at least another 30 minutes to complete the procedure.

Tourniquet pain is often the limiting factor in IVRA. It is difficult to manage, and with the remaining operative time, we need to use general anesthesia. Because instrumenting the airway is a major trigger for bronchospasm, the laryngeal mask airway (LMA) is probably a good choice in this setting.

We inform the patient she will be put to sleep for the remainder of the operation, to assure her comfort. We preoxygenate/denitrogenate with 100% oxygen by facemask, then induce with 200 mg propofol. We insert a #4 LMA with some difficulty. Within 2 minutes, spontaneous ventilation resumes with an end-tidal CO_2 of 45 mmHg. We continue propofol at 100 mcg/kg/min, with 50% N_2O in oxygen. Ten minutes before the end of the operation we give 3 mg of morphine i.v. to minimize early post-operative pain. Three minutes later her respiratory rate has increased to 30 breaths per minute, and the end-tidal CO_2 has fallen. Lung auscultation reveals bilateral wheezing.

Morphine can cause histamine release, inducing bronchospasm. We have several options for treatment. Volatile anesthetics are good bronchodilators, and can be used in the patient spontaneously breathing through an LMA. Halothane or sevoflurane are not pungent and work well as bronchodilators. However, halothane can sensitize the heart to the arrhythmogenic effects of sympathomimetic drugs. We use sevoflurane and do not hesitate to administer nebulized albuterol through the LMA, and, if all else fails, racemic epinephrine. A stethoscope would have allowed early detection of wheezing and perhaps prevention of full-blown bronchospasm.

In retrospect, if the surgeons suspected this may not be a straightforward carpal tunnel release, requiring more than 30–40 minutes, then a regional anesthetic (brachial plexus block) would have afforded a longer duration of action and probably avoided instrumentation of the airway. The mild local anesthetic toxicity could have been much worse with a complete failure of the tourniquet.

Emergence from anesthesia: During closure of the incision, we discontinue the anesthetic agents. When the bandage has been applied, we release the tourniquet and remove the LMA.

After an hour-long surgical procedure release of the tourniquet will not flood the system with local anesthetic and there is no longer risk of toxicity.

Post-anesthesia care: There should be little pain from this procedure. We leave the patient in the PACU with standing prn[1] orders of fentanyl for pain, rather than morphine, because of her bronchospastic reaction. We also write orders for an anti-emetic drug, should it be needed.

Discharge: When the patient is fully awake and tolerating oral intake, she can be discharged home with a caregiver, a prescription for an analgesic, and instructions not to drive for 24 hours.

NOTE

1. prn = *pro re nata*; as the need arises.

Cataract removal under MAC

The following case will describe the use of monitored anesthetic care (MAC).

Learning objectives:

- pre-operative management of the elderly patient
- methohexital
- oculo-cardiac reflex.

An 85-year old woman comes for removal of a cataract.

History. She has suffered significant visual loss from the cataract. Her past medical history reveals that she has given birth to four children and that she had an uncomplicated cholecystectomy under general anesthesia 40 years ago. She has no family history of anesthetic complications. She takes no medications, has no allergies and does not smoke. She drinks wine socially.

Physical examination reveals:

African American woman in no acute distress; weight 65 kg; height 5′2″ (155cm)
BP 150/90 mmHg; HR 90 beats/min; respiratory rate 16 breaths/min
Airway: Edentulous, Mallampati II, 4 fb mouth opening, 4 fb thyromental distance, full neck extension
CV: S1,S2 no murmur
Resp: Lungs clear to auscultation bilaterally

No additional preoperative laboratory or other studies are required in this ASA I patient.

Such minor eye procedures are usually performed under local anesthesia (peribulbar or retrobulbar) administered by the ophthalmologist. Injection of the local is not without pain, however transient, so we usually anesthetize the patient briefly (minutes).

Anesthetic preparation: We discuss the risks/benefits of the anesthetic plan, giving the patient an idea of what to expect: "You will be asleep for about 2 minutes while the surgeon places numbing medicine around your eye. After you wake up you will not be able to see as there will be a drape over your face. We will blow air under the drape and we will be monitoring your heart and lungs. You should feel no pain but let us know should you be uncomfortable or if you need to cough or move."

Induction of anesthesia: The eye block may be placed in the operating room, or in the preoperative holding area, allowing more time for it to take effect. Either way, we apply standard monitors, give the patient some supplemental oxygen, and then administer a short-acting induction agent such as methohexital (Brevital®) or thiopental. When the patient loses consciousness, the ophthalmologist places the block and tests it as soon as the patient awakens. Some patients become transiently apneic following the induction agent, and we need to support their airway (chin lift) or their ventilation with a mask until they resume spontaneous breathing.

Once the eye is anesthetized, the patient must remain still for some time. Because many patients will move as they doze off, following their brief anesthesia-induced respite, we administer no additional sedatives and the patient remains awake for the remainder of the procedure.

Maintenance of anesthesia: No additional sedatives are administered.

Complication: Suddenly the patient's heart rate falls to 30 beats/min and she complains of not feeling well.

The most likely culprit of sudden onset bradycardia in this setting is the oculocardiac reflex. Traction on the eye and ocular muscles can result in a slowing of the heart via a trigeminovagal pathway.[1] The bradycardia usually resolves immediately upon removal of the stimulus. The reflex response fatigues over time, but if it prevents progress of the operation, an anti-cholinergic may be required.

The ophthalmologist releases pressure on the eye, with immediate recovery of the heart rate to 70 beats/min. When the surgeon attempts to resume the operation, the heart rate again falls. After several attempts, we give glycopyrrolate 0.4 mg i.v. The patient's heart rate rapidly increases to 90 beats/min and the surgery proceeds.

For its lack of central effects we choose glycopyrrolate over atropine.

When the surgery is complete we take the patient to the PACU where she is monitored for surgical complications for a brief time, then discharged home with a companion.

Note

1. The full pathway is ciliary ganglion → ophthalmic division of trigeminal nerve → gasserian ganglion → main trigeminal sensory nucleus in the fourth ventricle → vagus nerve.

Cesarean section under regional anesthesia

The following case will emphasize regional anesthesia and obstetric issues.
   Learning objectives:
- reflux: risks, prevention
- physiology: fluid dynamics
- neuraxial anesthesia: technique, epidural hematoma risk, hypotension risk
- vasopressors: ephedrine vs. phenylephrine
- neuraxial opioids: pros/cons, risks.

A 28-year-old primiparous (first baby), pre-eclamptic woman requires a cesarean section for breech presentation of a 38-week fetus.

History. She had a normal prenatal course. This morning she complained of headache, blurred vision and swelling in her face, feet and hands. She is hypertensive, has proteinuria and generalized edema.

Her constellation of symptoms and findings suggest severe preeclampsia.[1] We need to control her blood pressure, start a magnesium infusion to reduce the risk of eclamptic seizure, and deliver the baby as soon as possible.

Review of systems: Reflux and low back pain with pregnancy.

These are normal findings in pregnancy. Progesterone-induced relaxation of the lower esophageal sphincter, increased acid secretion, and elevated intra-abdominal pressure increase the risk of aspiration of acidic gastric contents, a dangerous and potentially fatal complication during general anesthesia for delivery.

Physical examination: Anxious Caucasian woman in no distress; weight 100 kg; height 5'6"
(165 cm)
BP 160/110 mmHg; HR 100 beats/min; respiratory rate 18 breaths/min
Generalized edema including face
Airway: Mallampati I, 4 fb mouth opening, 4 fb thyromental distance, full neck extension
CV: S1, S2 no murmur
Respiratory: Lungs clear to auscultation, no râles
Neurologic: Reflexes 4+

To interpret these findings, we must recognize the normal physiologic changes of pregnancy:

- increased blood volume – plasma volume increases more than red blood cell mass leading to a dilutional anemia
- vasodilation to accommodate the increased volume
- increased respiratory drive – a central progesterone effect $\rightarrow$ a decrease in baseline $PaCO_2$ to 30 mmHg $\rightarrow$ increased minute ventilation. Surprisingly this is achieved mostly by increasing the tidal volume.

Pre-eclampsia reverses the gestational vasodilation leading to hypertension, and increases capillary permeability resulting in proteinuria, reduced intravascular volume, and cerebral, peripheral and potentially pulmonary edema.

Pre-operative studies: Urine protein dipstick 4+; hemoglobin 12 g/dL; hematocrit 36%; platelets 120 000/μL.

Pre-eclampsia can progress to *H*emolysis, *E*levated *L*iver enzymes, *L*ow *P*latelets (HELLP) syndrome. Therefore, before placing an epidural or spinal anesthetic we obtain a platelet count. A low platelet count would raise the specter of an epidural or subdural hematoma, a dreaded complication of neuraxial anesthesia. Proteinuria is routinely tested in pregnancy, and is one of the diagnostic criteria of pre-eclampsia.

Anesthetic preparation: We discuss the risks/benefits of regional vs. general anesthesia, she chooses regional. She drinks 15 mL of a non-particulate antacid (sodium citrate) just before moving back to the OR, where we keep her nerves in check with engaging conversation.

Anesthetic options in this ASA III patient include neuraxial anesthesia (spinal or epidural) or general anesthesia. We prefer regional anesthesia for several reasons: (i) all anesthetics that reach the brain also cross the placenta, therefore if the mother is asleep, we will deliver a drowsy baby, increasing the risk of neonatal depression; (ii) the mother (and often a companion) can witness the birth; and (iii) in most cases we have no need to manage her airway. The latter is particularly important in this population where the usual risks associated with general anesthesia are increased (inability to ventilate and/or intubate, aspiration of gastric contents). We explain the risks to the mother.

With an epidural, we avoid an all too rapid development of a sympathetic block and, with it, of hypotension in this hypovolemic patient. Because we do not routinely sedate these patients, reassuring conversation throughout the procedure is essential.

Establishment of regional anesthesia: We have the patient sit on the bed, attach standard monitors, and increase the flow rate of crystalloid (normal saline or Ringer's lactate) into her i.v. We gently place a lumbar epidural catheter and confirm that it is neither in a vein nor the intrathecal space (no change in hemodynamics or sensation following 3 mL of 2% lidocaine with 1:200 000 epinephrine). We then help the patient lie down with left uterine displacement, and dose the catheter with 5 mL aliquots of the same solution until a T4 level is attained or the maximum dose (7 mg/kg) is reached. Maternal blood pressure may require support as the epidural takes effect.

The fluid bolus should help offset the hypotension from sudden vasodilation, but must be administered with caution as this preeclamptic patient is prone to pulmonary edema. Pregnancy increases the risk of epidural vessel cannulation as these vessels dilate to provide collateral circulation around the compressed intra-abdominal vessels. We minimize this compression by either tilting the table to the left or placing a wedge under the right hip, which moves the uterus off the vena cava. If the patient is in labor, we test the catheter position between contractions to avoid pain-induced tachycardia masking a positive test dose. For blood pressure support, we prefer ephedrine in pregnancy. Phenylephrine may constrict the uterine vasculature and, in large doses, reduce perfusion. If instead she remains hypertensive, we choose labetalol or hydralazine to control her blood pressure.

Maintenance of anesthesia: Following delivery of the child, we start a pitocin infusion, administer prophylactic antibiotics, and inject morphine into the epidural catheter for post-operative pain management.
During uterine closure the patient complains of upper abdominal pain. We apply a face mask with 50% nitrous oxide in oxygen.

Neuraxial duramorph (long-acting morphine) has many side effects – particularly nausea, itching and (rarely) respiratory depression – but these are far outweighed by its benefits in reduced post-operative pain. Pitocin is routinely administered to increase uterine tone and reduce blood loss. It should be given as a rapid infusion as bolus-dosing can cause hypotension. Should the uterus remain atonic, the standard second-line agent, methergine (an ergot alkaloid), is avoided in the pre-eclamptic patient because it may exacerbate vasoconstriction and hypertension.

Nitrous oxide is a fair analgesic with minimal cardiovascular effects. Because MAC (minimum alveolar concentration) is reduced 40% in pregnancy, nitrous oxide gains in effectiveness.

Emergence from anesthesia: Following conclusion of the operation we try to remove the epidural catheter, but in our zest the catheter breaks.

Epidural catheters have great tensile strength, but even the toughest plastic is no match for the over-aggressive. If the catheter does not come out easily, we place the patient in the position in which the catheter was originally placed. Should a catheter break, we inform the patient that a small amount of the plastic tubing remains in her back, but should cause no problem in the future. The tip is radio-opaque and may show up on subsequent imaging.

Post-anesthesia care: The epidural level recedes over 2–3 hours. We continue intravenous fluids, pitocin and magnesium.

Common PACU problems include epidural-induced shivering (Rx: meperidine or tramadol), morphine-induced pruritus (Rx: nalbuphine (a mixed agonist-antagonist opioid)), nausea/vomiting (possibly morphine-induced, Rx: anti-emetics), pain (Rx: ketorolac (safe even with nursing), opioids).

Discharge: After we document that the block is receding, we discharge the patient to the ward for 2–3 days recuperation before letting her go home.

The neuraxial duramorph provides analgesia for 12–18 hours. Additional sedative or opioid analgesics during this time risk respiratory depression, but pain should be treated! Continuous monitoring by pulse oximetry enables early detection of respiratory depression – provided the patient does not receive supplemental oxygen.

NOTE

1. Severe pre-eclampsia is defined by, among other things, presence of headache and visual disturbance.

Gastric bypass under general anesthesia

Learning objectives:
- anesthesia for the morbidly obese patient
- obstructive sleep apnea
- fiberoptic intubation
- epidural anesthesia for post-operative pain.

A 40-year-old morbidly obese woman comes for a gastric bypass operation.

This intra-abdominal procedure involves restriction of the stomach to give the patient a sense of fullness even with limited oral intake. It may be performed by laparotomy or laparoscopy, and rarely involves significant blood loss.

History: She is morbidly obese despite multiple diets, one of which involved the drug Fen-Phen.

Use of Fen-Phen (fenfluramine–phentermine), a popular diet pill in the 1990s, has been blamed for the development of heart valve abnormalities and pulmonary hypertension.

Review of systems: Chronic hypertension; obstructive sleep apnea (OSA) requiring a CPAP mask at night; adult-onset diabetes mellitus; reflux; chronic low back pain.

We associate all of these finding and symptoms with morbid obesity. The OSA worries us in particular because of its association with pulmonary hypertension and difficult airway management.

Medications: Calcium-channel blocker, diuretic, oral hypoglycemic, H_2 blocker.

We will ask the patient to take her calcium-channel and H_2 blockers the morning of surgery, but neither the diuretic (she will already be dehydrated from her *n.p.o.* period) nor the oral hypoglycemic (without food intake, her blood sugar could fall dangerously low).

Physical examination: Morbidly obese Caucasian woman in no distress; weight 220 kg; height 5′ (150 cm)

BP 150/90 mmHg; HR 90 beats/min; respiratory rate 18 breaths/min
Airway: Mallampati IV; 3fb mouth opening; 4fb thyromental distance; full neck extension
CV: S1, S2 no murmur
Respiratory: Lungs clear to auscultation.

Obesity is an independent risk factor for difficult tracheal intubation. Though the majority of obese patients are easily intubated via direct laryngoscopy, presence of additional risk factors suggests the need for an awake intubation. Intravenous access may be difficult and various possible sites should be examined.

Pre-operative studies: Hgb 12 g/dL; Hct 36%; Plt 250 000/μL;
Na 140 mEq/L; K 4.2 mEq/L; BUN 23 mg/dL; Cr 1.3 mg/dL; glucose 105 mg/dL (5.2 mmol/L)
ABG : pH 7.40; pCO_2 40 mmHg; pO_2 95 mmHg; bicarbonate 28 mEq/L
ECG : normal sinus rhythm at 90 beats/min, ST segments at baseline
Echocardiogram: normal valves and pulmonary artery pressures

Infrequently, laparoscopic gastric bypass can result in significant blood loss, hence we like to know the starting hematocrit. Also, should that hematocrit be abnormally high, we will look even more closely at her pulmonary function (chronic hypoxemia-induced polycythemia?). We check her fasting blood glucose level because of her diabetes, and electrolytes because of her use of a diuretic. BUN and creatinine values can reveal renal insufficiency from diabetes and/or hypertension. Other studies further evaluate the impact of her OSA including the arterial blood gas (ABG), which shows no CO_2 retention, and the ECG, which shows no evidence of right ventricular hypertrophy.

Preparation for anesthesia. For post-operative pain management, we offer epidural anesthesia, placed awake with sedation carefully titrated to effect. She needs general endotracheal anesthesia. Because we worry about intubation of her airway, we plan an awake fiberoptic intubation and therefore give her glycopyrrolate.
We also order metoclopramide and bicitra.

Use of an epidural catheter for post-operative pain control in this setting (morbid obesity, incision near the diaphragm) can reduce the need for opiates and their antitussive effects and thus the threat of pulmonary complications. Sedation must be titrated to effect without compromising the patient's ventilation.

We facilitate fiberoptic visualization with an anti-sialogogue (glycopyrrolate) to dry secretions. Were she not already taking an H_2 blocker, we might add that to her preoperative medications, intended to reduce the risk of aspiration of gastric contents and its sequelae.

Induction of anesthesia. We place a thoracic epidural catheter under moderate sedation, encountering some (not unexpected) technical difficulty. Once placed and tested we move to the operating room.
After topical pharyngeal lidocaine, we perform superior laryngeal and transtracheal blocks. We smoothly advance a fiberoptic scope into her trachea and advance the endotracheal tube

without so much as a tiny gag. Once we detect end-tidal CO_2 on the capnograph, we induce general anesthesia with a small dose of thiopental and turn on the isoflurane vaporizer.

Obese patients challenge even the expert at placing epidural catheters. Persistence, a cooperative patient, and experience eventually win out. One useful trick: repeatedly ask the patient whether she feels the needle to the right or left of midline – sometimes finding the midline itself can be tricky.

Obese patients desaturate rapidly with apnea because of both a reduced functional residual capacity (FRC) and increased oxygen consumption. We have cause for concern, given the likely difficulty with mask ventilation (decreased chest wall compliance), potentially difficult tracheal intubation, and even a problem identifying tracheal rings should a surgical airway become necessary (heaven forbid!).

Maintenance of anesthesia. We maintain anesthesia with isoflurane in 50% inspired oxygen in air, titrating the volatile agent to maintain hemodynamic stability and a BIS (bispectral index) between 40 and 60. After the surgeon inflates her abdomen with carbon dioxide, she requires high peak inspiratory pressures (40–50 cm H_2O) to achieve an adequate tidal volume. Local anesthetics administered through the epidural catheter provide relaxation of her abdominal muscles, making the operation a little easier for the surgeon. A solid epidural block to the level of T5 also minimizes the need for volatile anesthetic agents. We re-dose the epidural with 2% lidocaine with 1:200 000 epinephrine every 60–90 minutes depending on the clinical situation.

After a lengthy operation, morbidly obese patients have a slow emergence from volatile anesthetics, which are highly soluble in the poorly perfused fat, forming a depot of anesthetics. We do not use nitrous oxide, which might expand gas in bowel and thus add difficulties for the surgeon. Obese patients may also have increased CNS sensitivity to medications, particularly opioids. The reliance on regional anesthesia reduces the need for both volatile agents and narcotics. We allow the epidural anesthetic to wane into analgesia (minimal or no motor block) before the procedure ends so she will be able to maintain her airway, breathe deeply and cough effectively upon extubation of her trachea.

Emergence from anesthesia. Following conclusion of the operation the patient awakens. She is strong, following commands, has a gag reflex and has a good respiratory pattern. We extubate her trachea and transport her to the PACU with the epidural infusion running for postoperative pain relief. We report to the PACU physician, including plans for postoperative pain management.

All patients should meet extubation criteria before the endotracheal tube is removed: fully awake, following commands, able to protect the airway, breathing spontaneously. Here we are particularly concerned because this patient was difficult to intubate. Therefore, we delay extubation several minutes (or longer), or use a "tube exchanger" – a long stylet that we place down the endotracheal tube, then leave in the trachea after extubation providing a conduit for reintubation should the need arise.

Post-anesthesia care. We manage her pain with the epidural infusion. Should she require additional analgesics, we should be extremely cautious with those that can depress ventilation.

Common PACU complications include desaturation, hypertension due to pain, and hypotension due to inadequate fluid replacement and/or epidural-induced sympathectomy. Trouble arises should a synergistic effect of weakened muscle power from the epidural block compound respiratory depression from narcotics.

PACU event – Desaturation. After about 30 minutes the nurse calls the PACU physician because the patient's SpO_2 has fallen below 90% despite 4 L/min oxygen via nasal cannula. She is arousable, after which her saturation improves temporarily, but declines again as she falls back asleep.

We consider the many etiologies of hypoxemia, and investigate the likelihood of each:
- *Narcosis*? She has received no intravenous opioids, and the concentration in the epidural infusion is unlikely to cause significant respiratory depression.
- *High epidural block with muscle weakness*? Her upper and lower extremities are strong – ruling out this diagnosis.
- *Residual neuromuscular blockade*? She did not receive any non-depolarizing muscle relaxants intraoperatively, relying instead on the epidural for relaxation.
- *Atelectasis*? Probably part of the problem, but would not explain desaturation only while asleep.
- *Obstructive sleep apnea*? This rises to the top of the list when we watch the patient breathe. She snores loudly and, though difficult to see but readily felt by placing a gentle hand over her larynx, a tracheal tug is evident with each inspiration. With some breaths she fails to move any air at all.

This patient requires CPAP to sleep at home. Lingering anesthetic effects and decreased afferent sensory input from the epidural anesthetic reduce stimulation to breathe, which might conspire with her upper airway pathology and thus worsen a sleep apnea. She requires CPAP. We keep the patient awake until a Respiratory Therapist brings the necessary equipment.

Discharge. After we confirm the epidural block is behaving as expected (return of muscle function but excellent analgesia), and are confident with her ventilation, we discharge the patient to the floor with continuous pulse oximetry. We alert the surgical service of her dependence on CPAP and the need for respiratory monitoring on the ward. We also inform the acute pain service (APS) of her location so they can manage her epidural medications for the next 2–3 days, until the pain level subsides and she is able to take oral medications.

In the post-operative orders we restrict additional opioids or sedatives except as prescribed by the Acute Pain Service. These members of the anesthesia care team will be available on call as needed and will see the patient on rounds at least twice daily to adjust dosing regimens and ensure safety.

AV shunt placement under peripheral nerve block

The following case will emphasize peripheral nerve block anesthesia and risks associated with care of the diabetic patient.

Learning objectives:
- anesthetic implications of chronic renal failure
- anesthetic implications of diabetes
- regional anesthesia of the upper extremity.

A 60-year-old man comes for placement of an AV (arterio-venous) fistula for dialysis.

An AV fistula is usually placed in the arm and takes less than 2 hours on average. We expect no significant blood loss.

History: The patient with long-standing insulin-dependent diabetes has developed progressive renal failure over the last several years, requiring peritoneal dialysis for the last 6 months (last dialysis was overnight).

A dialysis-dependent patient will have his electrolytes checked before the operation.

Review of systems: Chronic hypertension; diabetes, now with good control on insulin (HbA1c 6% last month); can walk 1 mile or climb a flight of stairs without chest pain; denies orthopnea or paroxysmal nocturnal dyspnea.

Diabetics are at risk of hypertension and chronic renal failure. Considering his risk for delayed gastric emptying, we insist that a diabetic patient remain *npo* after midnight. If not allowed to eat, his blood sugar may become dangerously low if he takes his morning insulin. Thus, we are very concerned with peri-operative control of his blood glucose, and therefore instruct him to take only half of his night-time dose of NPH, skip his morning insulin, and we schedule his operation early in the morning whenever possible. In the pre-operative holding area we check a "chem stick" (capillary blood glucose) before surgery and treat with insulin and/or glucose to maintain a level of 100 to 200 mg/dL ($\sim$6.0–12.0 mmol/L). If a delay occurs in his surgery time, we might have the patient report to preoperative holding early for blood glucose management. While his cardiac status appears good, and the

Cardiac Guidelines ("Eagle criteria") would not necessitate further evaluation, we might reasonably ask for a 12-lead ECG in the last 3 months, considering the risk of silent ischemia in hypertensive, diabetic patients.

Medications. Labetalol (for hypertension), insulin (NPH and regular), erythropoeitin (for anemia), Phoslo (to bind dietary phosphorus), calcitriol (to increase dietary calcium absorption and replace vitamin D).

This is basically a standard "laundry list" of medications for the ESRD patient. Considering his risk of a cardiac event, more aggressive beta blockade, to lower heart rate below 70 beats/min, is indicated in this ASA IV patient.

Physical examination: Moderately obese white man in no distress; weight 100 kg; height 5′10″ (175 cm);
BP 170/95 mmHg; HR 90 beats/min; respiratory rate 12 breaths/min
Airway: Mallampati II; 3fb mouth opening; 4fb thyromental distance; full neck extension
CV : S1, S2, no S3, S4 or murmur
Respiratory: lungs clear to auscultation
Neurologic: sensation intact in all extremities.

The risk of peripheral neuropathy in the long-standing diabetic looms large. Because we often use regional anesthesia for this operation and because regional anesthesia might be blamed for neurologic symptoms, we must obtain a baseline neurologic assessment and document any existing neurologic deficits. Had we heard râles during the pulmonary examination and suspected volume overload, a chest radiograph would have been in order.

Pre-operative studies: Hgb 12 g/dL; Hct 36%; Plt 300 000/μL; Na 145 mEq/L; K 3.6 mEq/L; glucose 110 mg/dL (6.1 mmol/L); Mg 1.7 mEq/L
ECG : NSR at 90 beats/min, normal intervals, ST segments at baseline.

Mild anemia commonly coexists with chronic renal failure.

Preparation for anesthesia. Following informed consent, we place an infraclavicular block pre-operatively in the "Block Room" under midazolam and fentanyl sedation. We use a stimulating needle to identify the nerve sheath, and inject 35 mL of 1.5% mepivacaine with 50 mcg clonidine without complications.

This anesthetic choice should provide surgical anesthesia of the forearm for 4–5 hours with continued analgesia. While we usually sedate patients for this procedure, the use of regional anesthesia will place less of a drug burden on the patient than general anesthesia would. Considering all the side effects of drugs, particularly when renal clearance is eliminated, a "minimalist" approach seems reasonable (though it should be noted that it has never been proven that regional anesthesia improves outcome over that of general anesthesia for these (or any) patients, except possibly for Cesarean delivery).

Confirmation of anesthesia. In the OR, we test the level of anesthesia by gently scratching the skin of descending dermatome levels.

Maintenance of anesthesia. With the help of a nasal cannula attached to a capnograph, we monitor respiratory rate, and administer oxygen to maintain a $SpO_2 > 95\%$. We titrate sedation to effect.

Intra-operative event – Hypertension: Approximately 45 minutes into the operation, the patient's blood pressure has climbed to 195/110 mmHg with a heart rate of 95 beats/min. He is arousable and complains of a mild headache, but is not anxious or in pain from the operation.

Intra-operative hypertension has a long differential diagnosis. Leading the list in this patient, who denies surgical pain and anxiety, are iatrogenic fluid overload and exacerbation of underlying chronic hypertension, probably from missing a dose of anti-hypertensive medication. Because he cannot respond to diuretics, fluid restriction, beta blockade with the desired reduction of heart rate and, if necessary vasodilation are the best temporary measures until dialysis can be performed post-operatively.

Emergence from anesthesia. We attempt to time our sedation in anticipation of the end of surgery. We transfer the patient to the PACU for monitoring. At least partial recession of the block should be documented before discharge. We tell the patient not to touch anything hot with the affected hand because temperature perception will be impaired longer than motor or sensory functions.

Open repair of an abdominal aortic aneurysm in a patient with coronary artery disease

The following case will emphasize the care of a patient with vascular disease for a major operation.

Learning objectives:

- pre-operative evaluation of the patient with cardiovascular disease
- cardiovascular physiology
- invasive hemodynamic monitoring
- intra-operative myocardial ischemia.

A 70-year-old man is scheduled for open repair of an abdominal aortic aneurysm.

Based on the shape of the aneurysm, he was unsuitable for an endovascular stent procedure. Instead, he requires a highly invasive, open intra-abdominal procedure that involves cross-clamping the aorta for a time, with substantial implications for blood pressure management and potential for uncontrolled blood loss.

History. The aneurysm has been followed for 3 years after detection during coronary angiography. Its diameter has increased recently by 10 mm, and requires repair.

The location and extent of the aneurysm determine the level of the aortic cross-clamp. We are particularly concerned with the relationship of the clamp to the renal arteries, as supra-renal clamping requires renal protective maneuvers such as administration of mannitol. High clamp location may also endanger perfusion of the lower 2/3 of the spinal cord, which is supplied by the artery of Adamkiewicz arising from the aorta somewhere between T8 and L4.

Review of systems: Chronic hypertension; myocardial infarction (MI) 3 years ago with subsequent 3 vessel coronary artery bypass graft (CABG); currently he has stable angina with exertion, but walks 1 mile three times per week without chest pain. History of congestive heart failure (CHF), last exacerbation 6 months ago, now without orthopnea.

A patient rarely has vascular disease in only one vessel and we worry about cerebral as well as more coronary arterial disease.

Medications: ACE inhibitor, beta-blocker, diuretic.

We will ask this ASA IV patient to discontinue the ACE inhibitor the day of surgery, but to take his diuretic and beta-blocker.

Physical examination. African American man in no distress; weight 90 kg; height 6′ (180 cm)
BP 160/90 mmHg (equal in both arms); HR 70 beats/min; respiratory rate 12 breaths/min
Airway: Mallampati II; 3fb mouth opening; 4fb thyromental distance; full neck extension
CV: S1, S2, no S3, S4 or murmur
Resp: Lungs clear to auscultation
Lower extremities: mild edema.

In patients with vascular disease, we check blood pressure in both arms because it can vary significantly between them. We accept the higher one.

Pre-operative studies. Hgb 15 g/dL; Hct 45%; Plt 300,000/μL; Na 140 mEq/L; K 4.2 mEq/L;
ECG: NSR at 90 beats/min, Q waves present in II, III and aVF; ST segments at baseline
Echo (6 months old): left ventricular ejection fraction 35% (normal >50%); decreased wall motion inferiorly; normal valves.

Not only would we like to know his starting hematocrit, we should insist on a "type and cross" for four units of blood for two reasons: first, because this procedure can result in significant blood loss and second, because this patient has a history of coronary artery disease and, in case of hemorrhage, we may need to increase his oxygen carrying capacity. Measurement of electrolyte levels is indicated in a patient taking diuretics, as these drugs can wreak havoc on the electrolyte balance. The presented cardiac evaluation suffices if we go by the "Eagle criteria." We might ask for a chest radiograph to rule out pulmonary edema if we are uncertain about the results of our auscultation of the lungs.

Preparation for anesthesia. We plan to use a combined epidural and general endotracheal anesthetic, placing the epidural catheter pre-operatively under sedation.
Because of his cardiac history and anticipated hemodynamic swings associated with aortic clamping and unclamping, we plan to place pressure catheters in a radial artery and pulmonary artery.

Epidural anesthesia may help us both as a means to buffer the wildly varying afterload from cross clamp application and removal (see below), and to improve postoperative pain management. While we worry that the anticoagulation required for this operation increases the risk of epidural hematoma, this complication occurs primarily at placement and removal of the catheter, neither of which we will do during the period of anticoagulation.

With the arterial catheter, we can monitor the blood pressure literally beat-by-beat. It also provides a conduit for repeated arterial blood gas and acid-base determinations. We can use the pulmonary artery catheter (PAC) to assess cardiac output and ventricular filling.

Induction of anesthesia. We place the arterial catheter awake with sedation and local anesthesia.

Before inducing general anesthesia, we dose the epidural catheter with 2% lidocaine with 1:200 000 epinephrine to obtain a T6 level.

Following pre-oxygenation, we induce the patient with fentanyl, etomidate, vecuronium, and esmolol. We successfully intubate the trachea with minimal hemodynamic swings. We place a PAC via the right internal jugular vein and record a wedge pressure of 15 mmHg and cardiac output of 5 liters/min.

We choose etomidate for induction because of its minimal cardiac depression, and employ fentanyl and esmolol to reduce the tachycardic response to direct laryngoscopy. Vecuronium has few side effects in the patient with normal hepatic and renal function.

The wedge pressure and cardiac output are in the expected range for this patient.

Maintenance of anesthesia. We maintain anesthesia with isoflurane in air enriched with 50% oxygen combined with a fentanyl infusion, titrating the isoflurane to keep hemodynamics stable, and the BIS between 40 and 60. We re-dose the epidural anesthetic every 60–90 minutes depending on the clinical situation.

Because the procedure requires an intra-abdominal approach, we avoid nitrous oxide. Isoflurane depresses the cardiovascular system so we give as little as possible, relying on the hemodynamic changes and a "depth-of-anesthesia monitor" to guide us. By using the epidural for operative anesthesia, we limit the requirement for both volatile anesthetic and muscle relaxants, but its effects on the sympathetic nervous system must be considered.

Intra-operative event – Cross-clamping of the aorta. In addition to the vasodilation obtained from the epidural-induced sympathectomy, we administer a vasodilator such as nitroglycerin before aortic cross-clamping. Infra-renal clamp placement confers less risk of kidney problems, but still warrants consideration of mannitol. Before the cross-clamp is placed, we administer heparin 5000 u i.v.

Cross-clamping the aorta causes a sudden increase in afterload, which often but not invariably dramatically increases the blood pressure. While the epidural can buffer the increase by vasodilating the splanchnic bed, we administer vasodilators to lower the blood pressure just before cross-clamping. An anticoagulating dose of heparin prevents thrombosis below the cross-clamp.

Intra-operative event – Removing the cross-clamp. We prepare by increasing venous capacitance with nitroglycerin, filling up this new capacity with i.v. fluids or blood. Immediately before removal of the clamp, we stop the nitroglycerin infusion, acutely decreasing venous capacitance. The resulting transient volume overload quickly dissipates following release of the cross clamp.

During the period of cross-clamp, veins distal to the clamp recoil, returning much of their blood to the heart. Subsequently, hypoxia causes both vasodilation (increasing venous capacity in this area) and the accumulation of many vasodilating and cardiac depressant metabolites. Thus, removal of the cross-clamp opens up this large vascular bed, causing a massive shift in blood volume. A major decrease in blood pressure may follow, unless we plan ahead to fill that space with additional fluid and/or blood.

Following removal of the cross clamp, we document the presence of distal pulses via Doppler, and administer protamine to reverse the anticoagulant effect of heparin. We might test the adequacy of reversal with an ACT.

Intra-operative complication – Ischemia. BP 90/50 mmHg; HR 110 beats/min; SpO_2 95%;
ST segments 3 mm downward sloping in V_5;
PCWP 20 mmHg; cardiac output 2.3 liters/min
Hemoglobin 7 g/dL.

The ST segment changes suggest ischemia, and increased PCWP indicates ventricular dysfunction and decreased compliance.

Management of ischemia. Transesophageal echocardiography: new anterolateral wall motion abnormality
We titrate esmolol to HR 70–80 beats/min and add a nitroglycerin infusion as tolerated. We begin to transfuse packed red cells.

Using transesophageal echocardiography, we look for regional wall motion abnormalities, ventricular volume and function. Treatment must improve the myocardial oxygen supply : demand balance by reducing heart rate and wall tension, increasing coronary perfusion pressure (diastolic blood pressure), and increasing oxygen carrying capacity. Normalization of the ST segments and PCWP indicate successful treatment.

Emergence from anesthesia. Following conclusion of the operation we leave the patient's trachea intubated and him sedated for transport to the Intensive Care Unit where weaning from mechanical ventilation would occur over a day or two.

Transport of the intubated patient requires manual ventilation and continuous monitoring. We also bring along the equipment necessary to ventilate his lungs in case the endotracheal tube becomes dislodged (mask, laryngoscope, extra ETT).

Though not necessary for this operation, with a suprarenal clamp endangering perfusion of the distal spinal cord, we might awaken the patient immediately post-operatively to document neurologic function of the lower extremities.

Trauma patient under general anesthesia

Learning objectives:
- anesthesia for the trauma patient
- fluid management
- increased intracranial pressure.

The Emergency Department calls regarding an approximately 40-year-old man who was thrown from his car during a traffic accident. He was briefly unconscious but soon regained consciousness and was clearly intoxicated. Abdominal ultrasound revealed a splenic injury; he has hematuria and multiple orthopedic injuries. While in the CT scanner, the patient became more somnolent and now has a Glasgow Coma Score (GCS, Table Tr 8.1) of 9 (Eyes:2, Verbal:3, Motor:4). The scan was aborted, and the patient transported directly to the trauma operating room. We alert all available staff to meet us there, and confirm the blood bank is readying 8 units of type-specific blood and 4 units of fresh frozen plasma.

This case presents an acute emergency, with imminent risk to life (or limb). We have little time for preoperative evaluation. In this patient, without family around, we have no history, nor any information on medications or allergies. We cannot obtain informed consent for the operation or anesthesia. In fact such a situation mandates that we proceed in an attempt to save the patient's life, even without consent. We must evaluate his status as rapidly as possible, and induce anesthesia such that the operation can begin.

Centers designated to receive trauma cases maintain a "trauma operating room," always set up with the necessary equipment including rapid infusion systems for warm intravenous fluids, various vascular access devices, airway management and pressure monitoring equipment, and a selection of vasopressors.

We must rely on astute observation and physical examination. The GCS score tells us he has suffered at least a moderate brain injury. A full body survey might reveal tell-tale scars of past operations, for instance a sternotomy scar from a coronary artery bypass graft, or a small lower abdominal scar from an appendectomy. Bruises suggest locations of impact and elicit concerns over specific injuries. For example bruising over the ribs might indicate fracture and potential for pneumothorax and contusion of heart or lungs.

Table Tr 8.1. Glasgow Coma Score. Scored between 3 (worst) and 15 (best); correlates with degree of brain injury: >12 mild; 9–12 moderate, <9 severe

Best eye response (4)
1. No eye opening
2. Eye opening to pain
3. Eye opening to verbal command
4. Eyes open spontaneously

Best verbal response (5)
1. No verbal response
2. Incomprehensible sounds
3. Inappropriate words
4. Confused
5. Orientated

Best motor response (6)
1. No motor response
2. Extension to pain
3. Flexion to pain
4. Withdrawal from pain
5. Localizing pain
6. Obeys commands

Physical examination in the OR: Assessment of the ABCs (airway, breathing and circulation) takes precedence. We find him breathing with good air movement, reeking of alcohol, with a thready, rapid pulse. On more thorough examination we find:

Caucasian man of average build with obvious superficial trauma to face, chest, arms and legs with numerous scrapes; hard cervical collar in place; weight ~70 kg; height ~6′ (180 cm); bilateral chest tubes to water seal

BP 90/50 mmHg; HR 135 beats/min; respiratory rate 28 breaths/min

Airway: patient uncooperative, difficult to fully assess; 4fb thyromental distance; in hard cervical collar

CV: S1, S2 no murmur, tachycardic

Respiratory: Lungs clear to auscultation bilaterally

Neurologic: somnolent, moving all extremities, withdraws to pain, pupils equal and responsive to light

Access: 18 g intravenous catheter in right antecubital fossa, right subclavian double-lumen catheter.

This patient has suffered multiple traumatic injuries. To get a handle on where we stand we need to ask more questions of the surgeons, while simultaneously applying monitors.

Further history: He has an open left femur fracture; hematuria inferring kidney, ureter or bladder injury; free fluid in the abdomen suggesting hemorrhage from spleen, liver or intestines; multiple rib fractures but no evidence of pneumothorax; no obvious cervical spine fracture on X-ray or CT; and a small right temporal epidural hematoma on head CT. Chest tubes were placed on arrival in the Emergency Department because of apparent rib fractures, subsequently a subclavian catheter was inserted. He received a total of 4L Ringer's lactate, 2 units Type O+, uncrossmatched blood and 3 mg i.v. morphine in the Emergency Department.

Laboratories and studies (from 30 min prior, before blood administered):

Hgb 9 g/dL; Hct 27%; Plt 150 000/μL;

Na 140 mEq/L; K 3.9 mEq/L; BUN 12 mg/dL; Cr 0.8 mg/dL; glucose 165 mg/dL (8.2 mmol/L)

PT and aPTT: pending

Blood type: A$^+$.

This additional history adds to our concern. The issues with which we wrestle include the following:

- *Airway management* We cannot rule out the presence of cervical spine instability or injury. Static radiographs cannot evaluate the quality of the ligaments that protect the cervical spinal cord from damage during head movement as in traditional laryngoscopy. We consider all trauma patients to have a full stomach, with risk of regurgitation and aspiration of gastric contents. Standard application of cricoid pressure, a mainstay of aspiration prophylaxis, can displace a fractured cervical spine potentially compressing the spinal cord. In the patient with spinal cervical injury we support the posterior neck while compressing the cricoid ring, either with bi-manual pressure or taking advantage of the posterior portion of the hard cervical collar. Unfortunately that collar, with its bulk, proximity, and interference with mouth opening, makes management of the airway difficult.

- *Intravascular volume status* We find accurate assessment of volume status difficult. Significant blood can be lost into concealed spaces such as the thigh and abdomen. If the abdomen is tense, the high pressure might curtail intraabominal bleeding. Upon opening of the tight abdomen, a deluge of blood might signal the release of the tamponade. Establishing appropriate vascular access should be a high priority. In the presence of abdominal trauma, vascular access must be sought in the upper body, as products administered through the femoral route, for example, might be lost into the abdomen en route to the central circulation. When the existing access is of inadequate caliber, as is often the case, we can supplement it with additional catheters, or consider exchanging one of the catheters over a wire (insert a long wire through the catheter, remove the catheter, then advance a new, more appropriate catheter over the wire). Fluid management should include consideration of hemoglobin concentration, electrolytes, and osmolality (Ringer's lactate is hypotonic). Decreasing plasma osmolality contributes to brain swelling.

- *Pulmonary status* Presence of rib fractures introduces the likelihood of pneumothorax and/or pulmonary contusion. While not apparent on an initial chest radiograph, decreasing pulmonary compliance with positive pressure ventilation (increasing peak inspiratory pressure) could herald the development of a pneumothorax, which should be noted and treated right away, before becoming a tension pneumothorax.
- *Cardiovascular status* With no knowledge of any pre-existing cardiovascular disease, we must focus on his current state. The hypotension and tachycardia are most likely a function of his hypovolemia, but other causes must be considered. High on the list would be cardiac tamponade or contusion, tension pneumothorax (if a chest tube is malfunctioning), fat embolism from the femur fracture, transfusion reaction, anaphylaxis, spinal shock, and electrolyte abnormalities (especially calcium from massive blood transfusion).
- *Neurologic status* The fact the patient was conscious at the scene gives reason to hope for a reasonable neurologic outcome, but his state is becoming grave. With hypotension and likely increasing intracranial pressure (ICP), we must concern ourselves with cerebral perfusion.[1] The neurosurgeon will place an ICP monitor, allowing calculation of the CPP. In the meantime, increasing blood pressure takes precedence; we also consider measures to reduce the ICP including hyperventilation, mannitol, avoiding a head-down position, e.g., Trendelenburg's position, administering no hypotonic fluids and avoiding those with glucose. Once a ventriculostomy has been placed, we can easily reduce the CSF volume, and better monitor the actual CPP.

Preparation for anesthesia. We talk to the patient reassuringly as we connect our standard monitors and begin pre-oxygenation. We loosen his cervical collar sufficient to view the trachea, while an assistant prepares the patient's right wrist for a radial arterial catheter.

In trauma cases such as this we exercise our resource management skills and encourage "parallel processing." We orchestrate several helpers performing simultaneous procedures, to facilitate a rapid beginning of the operation(s).

Despite his altered mental status we continue to speak to the patient as we would want our loved ones spoken to in a similar situation.

Induction of anesthesia. Following adequate de-nitrogenation, we induce anesthesia with etomidate 21 mg (~0.3 mg/kg), fentanyl 100 mcg and succinylcholine 70 mg (~1 mg/kg). One assistant provides in-line stabilization of the spine without traction, and another applies bimanual cricoid pressure, while we perform a gentle direct laryngoscopy and advance an 8.0 mm endotracheal tube through the vocal cords. After confirming the presence of end-tidal CO_2, we secure the tube and begin mechanical ventilation with a rate of 15 breaths/min and a tidal volume of 600 mL, titrated to an end-tidal CO_2 of 25 mmHg.

We prefer a rapid sequence induction because of aspiration risks, but find pros and cons to all available agents. We wish to limit the systemic response to intubation, reduce ICP, decrease the cerebral metabolic rate for oxygen ($CMRO_2$), while avoiding hypotension. In the presence of hypovolemia, cardiovascular depression from thiopental and propofol can cause hypotension. Though often considered the preferred agent in hypovolemia due to its stimulation of the sympathetic nervous system, ketamine increases ICP and is therefore relatively contraindicated in this case. Etomidate usually causes little change in the blood pressure, and reduces $CMRO_2$, but can result in a hypertensive response to intubation. For muscle relaxation we prefer succinylcholine for a rapid-sequence induction, particularly when the airway examination is less than optimal. Should intubation of the patient's airway prove difficult, the paralysis will last only a few minutes, then spontaneous respiration should resume. Though succinylcholine can cause a small, transient increase in ICP, we can blunt the effect with an adequate induction agent and/or hyperventilation. The non-depolarizing muscle relaxant alternatives do not possess the rapid onset and offset of succinylcholine, but become useful in patients at risk for hyperkalemia (burns, crush injuries) or malignant hyperthermia.

We begin hyperventilation after conferring with the neurosurgeon, who also requests mannitol.

Induction of anesthesia, continued. During the induction, an assistant placed a right radial arterial catheter for continuous blood pressure measurement. While the general surgeon prepares and drapes the abdomen, another assistant sterilely places a 9-french "Swan Introducer" catheter into the left subclavian vein. All fluids are attached through warming circuits. We draw blood for arterial blood gas, electrolytes, hemoglobin and platelet concentrations. We transduce the arterial and central venous catheters: ABP 85/45 mmHg; HR 140 beats/min; CVP 2 mmHg.

By having an assistant place catheters, we free our hands for induction and maintenance of this critically ill patient. We choose the subclavian over internal jugular route for vascular access to avoid any impairment to cerebral venous drainage in this head-injured patient. The presence of chest tubes reduces the risk of complication from inadvertent pleural puncture. We send blood for analysis of hematocrit to gauge the resuscitation and determine needs for future blood products, as these take time to acquire from the blood bank.

Maintenance of anesthesia. We maintain anesthesia with judicious administration of opioids and isoflurane as tolerated in 50% inspired oxygen in air. We titrate the oxygen concentration to a saturation >95%, and the volatile agent to maintain hemodynamic stability. Before the surgeon opens the abdomen, we administer a non-depolarizing muscle relaxant and prepare for rapid infusion of fluids and blood should the blood pressure suddenly fall.

For abdominal operations we tend to avoid nitrous oxide for its propensity to increase the volume of air-containing spaces. With vasopressors in hand and ample vascular access, we are prepared for the abdomen to be opened.

Intra-operative event – Surgical incision. Upon opening the abdomen, the blood pressure falls precipitously as several liters of blood are evacuated. We rapidly infuse normal saline and begin infusing blood (already checked by nurses as to blood type and patient). We ask the nurse to order more blood and fresh frozen plasma from the blood bank. The Hemocue® (β-hemoglobin photometer) reads 7.2 g/dL. The surgeon identifies a splenic rupture and successfully clamps the supplying artery. We continue to administer blood based on the results of our laboratory and Hemocue® evaluations.

Meanwhile the neurosurgeon performs a small frontal craniotomy, draining about 75 mL blood, then places an ICP monitor so that the CPP can be kept at 70–90 mmHg.

With the bleeding apparently stopped and the hemodynamics stabilized at 110/60 mmHg with a heart rate of 90 beats/min and a CVP of 8 mmHg, the surgeon closes the abdomen to make room for the orthopedic surgeon to work on the femur fracture. Suddenly the blood pressure plummets again.

Careful evaluation of the findings can narrow the numerous potential causes for hypotension in this setting. An increased central venous pressure might accompany cardiac contusion, ischemia, tamponade, pulmonary embolism, or tension pneumothorax, the latter associated with increased peak inspiratory pressures during mechanical ventilation. Abdominal bleeding can be ruled out by direct inspection. Continued hemorrhage concealed in the pelvis, retroperitoneal space or thigh cannot be similarly ruled out, but should not cause such sudden instability.

We place a transesophageal echo (TEE) probe and find the right side of the heart virtually empty, and a fluid-density mass compressing the right ventricle. We diagnose cardiac tamponade and the surgeon proceeds to insert a needle into the pericardial sac, draining the pericardial blood with rapid improvement in venous return as observed by TEE. But the hypotension does not resolve completely, and the ventricle appears somewhat globally hypokinetic, we check electrolyte levels and find a potassium of 4.5 mEq/L and an ionized calcium of only 0.80 mmol/L (normal 1.03–1.30). The blood pressure responds to calcium infusion.

The femur fracture repair proceeds with much less fanfare.

When the cause of hypotension remains unclear, transesophageal echocardiography might prove helpful, as it did in this case. With massive transfusion, resulting hypocalcemia can depress cardiac contractility, and electrolyte levels should be assessed frequently. A word of warning, calcium drives potassium intracellularly (part of its role in treating hyperkalemia); thus a patient with hypokalemia can be pushed into ventricular fibrillation with rapid infusion of calcium. The lesson – do not rapidly administer calcium without first knowing the potassium level.

Emergence from anesthesia. Following conclusion of the operation we leave the patient paralyzed and sedated with his trachea intubated for transport to the Intensive Care Unit. He will suffer major fluid shifts over the next few hours, with possible pulmonary edema and airway swelling. Furthermore his neurologic status is unclear. The sedative and paralytic drugs will be discontinued to allow assessment of his neurologic status in the ICU.

Transport of this patient requires manual ventilation with a Mapleson system and oxygen source, and continuous monitoring. We bring along equipment to reintubate his trachea, should that become necessary; we have at hand the vasoactive agents we have required recently. In the ICU we give report, including updates on laboratory values, to the nurse and physician. We remind them the replaced subclavian catheter has not been radiographically evaluated, nor has the cervical spine been medically cleared.

We return to follow-up on the patient several times over the ensuing weeks. Expected to make a full recovery eventually, he is discharged to a rehabilitation center after three weeks.

NOTE

1. Cerebral perfusion pressure (CPP) is calculated as mean arterial pressure minus ICP or CVP, whichever is greater. We consider 60–80 mmHg an adequate CPP.

Index of select tables and figures